KU-751-148

THE *DASH* DIET

Lower your blood pressure in just 21 days

PRIYA TEW

aster

An Hachette UK Company
www.hachette.co.uk

First published in Great Britain
in 2020 by Aster, an imprint of
Octopus Publishing Group Ltd,
Carmelite House, 50 Victoria
Embankment, London EC4Y 0DZ

www.octopusbooks.co.uk
www.octopusbooksusa.com

Text copyright © Priya Tew 2020
Design and layout copyright ©
Octopus Publishing Group 2020

Distributed in the US by
Hachette Book Group,
1290 Avenue of the Americas,
4th and 5th Floors,
New York, NY 10104

Distributed in Canada by
Canadian Manda Group,
664 Annette St, Toronto,
Ontario, Canada M6S 2C8

All rights reserved. No part of this work
may be reproduced or utilized in any
form or by any means, electronic or
mechanical, including photocopying,
recording or by any information storage
and retrieval system, without the prior
written permission of the publisher.

Priya Tew asserts the moral right to be
identified as the author of this work.

ISBN 978-1-78325-406-4

A CIP catalogue record for this book
is available from the British Library.

Printed and bound in the UK.

10 9 8 7 6 5 4 3 2 1

All reasonable care has been
taken in the preparation of this
book but the information it
contains is not intended to take
the place of treatment by a
qualified medical practitioner.

Before making any changes in
your health regime, always consult
a doctor. While all the therapies
detailed in this book are completely
safe if done correctly, you must seek
professional advice if you are in any
doubt about any medical condition.
Any application of the ideas and
information contained in this book
is at the reader's sole discretion
and risk.

Commissioning Editor: Natalie Bradley
Senior Editor: Leanne Bryan
Copy Editor: Anne Sheasby
Senior Designer: Jaz Bahra
Typesetter: Jeremy Tilston
Senior Production Manager:
  Caroline Alberti

The FSC® label means that materials
used for this product have been
responsibly sourced.

MIX
Paper from
responsible sources
FSC® C104740

To my three children, Kezia, Judah and Etty,
who patiently played and let me write this
through lockdown.

Thank you for believing in me and
cheering me on.

Cook's notes

Some general guidance for the recipes in this book.

- Standard level spoon measurements are used in all recipes.
- 1 tablespoon = 15ml.
- 1 teaspoon = 5ml.
- Eggs should be medium-sized unless otherwise stated.
- Fruit and vegetables should be medium-sized unless otherwise stated.
- The weights given for all wholegrains are uncooked weights.
- All microwave information is based on an 800-watt oven. Follow the manufacturer's instructions for an oven with a different wattage.

Contents

Introduction

It may have 'diet' in its name, but the DASH Diet is most certainly not another fad diet. It is a scientifically sound way of life that will benefit your heart, lower your blood pressure and help your whole family improve their health. Your blood pressure is how hard your blood is pushing against the artery walls.[1] Nearly 90 per cent of adults are likely to develop high blood pressure during their lifetime, which carries an increased risk of heart disease and stroke.[2] Only around 35 per cent of those with high blood pressure have it well controlled, so there is definitely room for improvement – and you can improve your own at home without medication.[3]

Our story starts in the 1990s, when researchers noted that people following a vegetarian/vegan diet had lower blood pressure. They set up a research trial to test out their hypothesis: would eating a diet higher in plant foods reduce blood pressure? The team compared a diet high in fruit and vegetables to a specialist diet they created, and this specialist diet became the DASH diet. The DASH trial (Dietary Approaches to Stop Hypertension) found that eating a diet high in fruits, vegetables and wholegrains, with a decent

1

helping of lean protein and a side of low-fat dairy, really did reduce people's blood pressure. This is the basis of the DASH diet. Now, some of this really isn't rocket science – it is common knowledge that fruit and vegetables are good for us. What makes the DASH diet different is the combination of foods and the portions. With plant-based eating on the rise, and with meat having the highest environmental impact of all foods, the DASH diet just makes good sense. While not being a restrictive diet, it does reduce your intake of red meat, salt, saturated fat and added sugars. It is now one of the most studied diets, with gold-standard scientific research to back it up. It was named by the British Dietetic Association as one of the few diets that actually do work, and is now included in several clinical guidelines across the globe.[4] It's a way of eating that really makes sense.

As a dietitian, I'm not normally someone who promotes diets – in fact, I shy away from the word. Why? Well, let's face it, most diets are fads and do not work long term. When you hear the word 'diet', it is usually associated with a restrictive way of eating that leads to the quick shedding of a few pounds in time for the summer or a special occasion or holiday. I'm afraid if that is what you are looking for, then you have not picked up the right book. Dietitians are trained in using therapeutic diets: diets for certain medical conditions that have to be scientifically researched and proven to work. The DASH diet is one of these. It is based on sound research, which has been proven time and time again. We know that if you follow this way of eating, you can lower your blood pressure, lower your cholesterol and improve your overall heart health. You may also find it helps in cases of type 2 diabetes – and it could help you lose weight.

The Western diet has changed a lot over the past 50 years, moving from home-cooked food with more plants to a lot of animal-based, high-fat, high-sugar, processed, pre-made foods. We have also become a lot less active and many of us have sedentary jobs. Eating habits during the Second World War, when people were on rations, included a lot more fruit and veg, and less meat and sugar. While we would not want to go back to that time and live through another world war, there is something to be said for simple eating, growing your own food and cooking from scratch. Dietary change and becoming more active could lead to substantial changes to your health and lower your risk of chronic diseases, such as cancer, heart disease and obesity. What would your usual food diary show us? Would it contain a lot of pre-bought convenience foods, salty foods, and high levels of sugar and animal fats? You would not be in the minority if so. Or would it be full of fruit and vegetables, wholegrains, plenty of plant proteins and healthy fats?

1
Hypertension & the Heart

Over the past 50–80 years, our diet and lifestyle has moved away from home-grown, home-cooked meals to convenience foods and a diet high in saturated fats, refined white carbohydrates and lots of snack foods. Our portion sizes have also increased, while our activity levels have decreased, with increasing numbers of desk jobs and more machines to do jobs for us. These are some of the reasons our risk of heart disease has increased.

Nowadays, heart disease is one of the main causes of death and disability in the UK, and one of the leading causes of death in the world. An estimated 2,000 people die of heart disease each day in the US, and it makes up 30 per cent of all global deaths.[1,2,3] The British Heart Foundation highlights that 7.4 million people in the UK are living with cardiovascular disease, costing the health service an estimated £9 billion each year. In a single day, it is the cause of death for 460 people.[4] With numbers this high, it makes sense that it's an area on which scientists have chosen to focus a lot of research.

Heart disease and stroke are the leading cause of death in the UK, killing one person every eight minutes, so you can see why it is key that we do something to help our bodies out. It has been said that any decrease in blood pressure will bring benefits (unless you have been diagnosed with low blood pressure), so there is huge motivation to make some lifestyle changes.

Reducing the risk of cardiovascular disease (including heart disease and stroke) will hopefully lead to people living longer, healthier lives. The good news is there are changes you can make to help reduce the risks. Physical inactivity, smoking, excess alcohol and a diet high in sodium and low in potassium (high in salt, low in fruit and veg) are all factors that increase the risk of heart disease and stroke – but they are also all things you can change!

When it comes to looking after your heart, or indeed your body in general, educating yourself on the risks can be a great motivator. Let's take a look at the risks and reasons you may have been drawn to this book in the first place.

Cardiovascular disease

Cardiovascular disease (CVD) is a general term for conditions that affect the heart or blood vessels. These can include coronary heart disease, stroke and blockages in the arteries on the arms/legs. Think about having a blocked drain: unless you look after your sink well over time, a build-up of grime stops the water from flowing as effectively. But if you clean it regularly, remove the debris from the plughole and are careful what you send down the sink, you are less likely to get a blockage. Similarly, in the body, you can get a build-up of fatty deposits in the arteries (known as atherosclerosis) that reduce the blood flow, while a larger blood clot could completely stop the flow of blood to the heart, limbs or brain. Looking after your body by making certain changes can help keep the blood at the right consistency and help prevent debris building up in the arteries.

How do we keep the blood flowing freely around the body?

Lifestyle changes, including your diet, can play a major role. This is where the DASH diet comes in. High blood pressure is the leading cause of CVD, with high cholesterol levels not far behind.[5] The research tells us that the DASH diet not only decreases blood pressure, but can also decrease our cholesterol levels. Addressing both of these factors simultaneously has great benefits for our cardiovascular health.[6]

Hypertension (or high blood pressure)

As I have explained, blood pressure measures how hard your blood is pushing against your artery walls.[7] High blood pressure, also known as hypertension, is a condition where your heart has to work extra hard to pump blood around the body.[8] It affects about 26 per cent of adults in the UK, increasing the risk of heart disease, heart failure, stroke and kidney disease.[9, 10]

Hypertension is when your blood pressure is between 140/90mmHg and 180/120mmHg.

140

The top number is your systolic pressure. This is the pressure in your blood vessels when your heart contracts and squeezes the blood out.

90 mmHg

The bottom number is your diastolic blood pressure. This is the pressure between heartbeats, when your heart is at rest and fills with blood.

$$\frac{150}{90}$$

If your blood pressure gets extremely high, you may get symptoms including dizziness and vision problems.

$$\frac{140}{90}$$

$$\frac{120}{80}$$

If your blood pressure gets too low, you may feel light-headed and dizzy.

$$\frac{90}{60}$$

With hypertension, your heart has to work harder to pump the blood around your body. This force can cause damage to the arteries and harden them. It could be that there is a blockage in an artery or the arteries have narrowed. Either way, this can put a strain on your heart and put you at risk of a heart attack or stroke. It also puts you at risk of damage to the blood vessels in your kidneys and eyes. The higher your blood pressure, the higher the risk.[11] Pretty scary facts.

Strokes and Usual BP

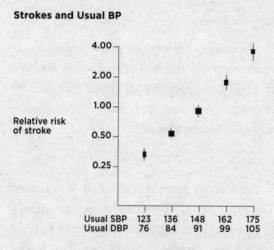

Figure 1. Stroke and usual blood pressure (BP) graph showing how the risk of stroke increases as your blood pressure increases.[12] Systolic blood pressure (SBP) is the pressure when the heart contracts, and diastolic blood pressure (DBP) is the pressure when the heart relaxes.

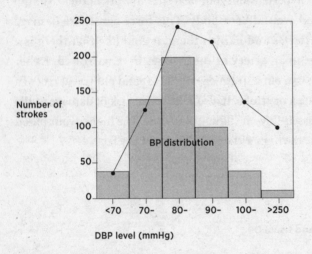

Number of strokes attributable to BP in population

Figure 2. Absolute number of strokes in 405,000 individuals in seven prospective observational studies by baseline diastolic blood pressure (DBP). Approximately three-quarters of all strokes attributable to blood pressure occurred among individuals classified as 'normotensive'.[13]

Unfortunately, there aren't general symptoms or warning signs to look out for to tell if your blood pressure slightly increases. Many people have high blood pressure but are unaware of it – it has been termed a 'silent killer'. This is why it is important your blood pressure is checked regularly when you visit your doctor.

If you are taking certain medications, it is even more important, as some medications can affect your blood pressure. A single blood pressure reading does not give an accurate picture, so your doctor may want to look at the pattern over a few readings. It can sometimes be necessary to measure your blood pressure over a 24-hour period using a portable instrument.

Our blood pressure varies over the course of a day: it will be lower when you relax and sleep, and will increase when you are active. Stress, anxiety and fear will also increase your heart rate. Your blood pressure will also naturally increase as you age. These variations are not a problem; the issue we are concerned about here is having high levels over a prolonged period of time. When your blood pressure is consistently high, it can damage your blood vessels and increase your health risks. In the long term, having high blood pressure can increase your risk of heart disease, and can also damage your kidneys, your eyes and the circulation in your legs. Treatment with diet, lifestyle and medication (if recommended by your doctor) can help.

What causes high blood pressure?

Sometimes the reasons for high blood pressure are unknown (essential hypertension). It can be a result of kidney disease, or the overproduction of certain hormones (secondary hypertension). Often, there may be no specific cause for your blood pressure being higher. It could be due to a medication you have been on, such as birth control pills, or it could be genetic. Whatever the reason, it is a good idea to focus on improving your nutrition and being active in your daily life.

Cholesterol

Cholesterol is often seen as the bad guy in terms of heart health, but it actually plays many important roles in the body, including making up part of cell membranes and helping the body to make hormones, vitamins and bile acids. It's not actually a 'bad fat' – we all need a certain level of it. Once again, it all comes down to balance.

Cholesterol is a type of fat found in the bloodstream and in the fatty outer layer of our cell membranes. It is transported around the body attached to proteins, and this whole combination of fat plus protein makes up lipoproteins. You can think of these lipoproteins as taxis. We have two taxi companies: one is HDL (high density lipoprotein), and the other is LDL (low density lipoprotein). The HDL taxis can only transport the 'good' cholesterol, while the LDL taxis are only able to transport what is often called the 'bad' cholesterol. In fact, we need both LDL and HDL in the body, but too high a level of LDL is not good for our heart health.

The role of the LDL taxi is to deliver cholesterol through the bloodstream to the tissues that need it. The problem comes when we have too high an amount. Too many LDL taxis will cause a traffic jam. In the body, too much LDL leads to fatty plaques in the arteries. These can cause a blockage, stopping the blood from being able to flow easily. This means there is more chance of a blood clot and a heart attack or stroke. You can see why we don't want too much LDL cholesterol around. Our HDL taxis are very different, as they actually go around picking up any LDL they see and taking it to the liver to be disposed of. So our HDL cholesterol has a protective effect on heart health.

The question is, how do we get the cholesterol balance right, with less of the LDL and more of the HDL? The main guidelines tell us to change our lifestyles. Exercise regularly, stop smoking, moderate your intake of alcohol and eat a healthy diet that contains less saturated fat. Saturated fats are the animal fats that are mainly found in red meat, butter, cheese, cream, cakes, biscuits, confectionery and takeaway meals. The DASH diet, with its focus on plants and cooking from scratch, will help you swap saturated fats for heart-healthier fats, such as olive oil and oily fish.

As nutrition is a pretty new science, we are constantly learning and evolving our thinking as new research is done. Over 20 years ago, it was thought that eggs should be avoided as they contain cholesterol. You would have been told to keep to just a couple of eggs a week. We now have longer-term research that shows the cholesterol in the egg is actually broken down and reused by the body to make whatever is needed, so eating cholesterol does not necessarily increase your cholesterol levels. While eating eggs daily could cause a small increase in LDL cholesterol, this is minimal – and, more importantly, eating eggs could also increase the beneficial HDL cholesterol levels in your body, which is helpful. This shows how important it is to keep up to date with research, to look in depth at what it says and not to take media headlines out of context. Eggs are highly nutritious, providing the body with zinc, iodine, iron and protein. Although they contain cholesterol and a little saturated fat, the conclusion is that eggs can definitely be part of a healthy, balanced diet. There is no set limit on how many you can eat, but as we want a variety of proteins in the diet, one to three a day seems sensible.

2

The DASH Diet:
An Overview

The DASH diet is not a diet, but a way of eating that embraces more plants, less saturated fat and less salt. It is rich in vitamins, minerals, antioxidants and fibre. If vegetarian/vegan populations tend to have lower blood pressure, does this mean we should stop eating meat? Well, there's more to it than that. Instead of cutting out foods from our diets, I think we need to be looking at what to eat more of, mainly plant foods. You can see the DASH diet as an extension of general healthy eating guidelines. In the UK, the government guidance for healthy eating is the Eat Well Plate. This model aims to encourage the whole population to eat more plants and less meat, which is known to be a more sustainable way of eating. The DASH diet helps us to do this, and there is something in this combination of foods and mix of nutrients that is protective against many diseases.

Eating the DASH way means you will eat plenty of fruits and vegetables, combined with low-fat dairy, wholegrains, beans and pulses, along with lean meat, poultry and fish, plus some servings of nuts and seeds. This is not something to try for a few weeks or months: it is a guide to changing your eating habits for life, to give your body the nutrients it needs to fight chronic diseases like heart disease. Of course, nutrition alone will not keep your body healthy throughout life, but it does play a vital role. There can be genetic factors that make you more likely to get ill, and environmental factors that you may not be able to change. Focusing on what you *can* change can help you feel like you are really doing something to help yourself. Alongside diet in this book, we will cover other lifestyle factors, including stress, exercise, motivation and sleep habits. By following these tips, I hope you will gain an improved sense of wellbeing and happiness, as well as lower blood pressure.

Current research suggests that the DASH diet can often lower blood pressure as much as medication can. You may be on medication (or have been offered medication) to help with your blood pressure, and this may be necessary. The information in this book is no substitute for advice from a healthcare professional/doctor who has you and your whole medical history in front of them. If you want to step away from using medication to control your blood pressure, always discuss that with your healthcare team first. If you have only just been diagnosed with high blood pressure, you may be able to try lifestyle changes first, then review and add in medications if these changes have not had enough of an effect. Or it could be that, while you may want to stay away from medication, your blood pressure is too high (180/120mmHg) and medication is needed to start with. Some people will need specialist treatment and medication alongside the DASH diet.[1] It could also be that, after changing your lifestyle for a period of time, you can adjust your medication. This must, of course, always be done with your doctor's supervision.

Who will benefit the most from the DASH diet?

The greatest benefits of the DASH diet may be for those with pre-hypertension (120–139/80–89mmHg). So if your blood pressure is just slightly high, then now is the right time to be making the changes outlined in this book. Hang on, I know what you are thinking: if I don't see my doctor regularly, then how will I know my blood pressure is on the rise? Well, you may not know, but as this way of eating and living is beneficial to all of us, it can also be a preventative measure. So, if you are concerned about high blood pressure, heart disease and stroke, then jump on board now.

It has long been recommended that the first line of treatment for high blood pressure is lifestyle change. A healthy diet and regular exercise can reduce blood pressure, but what exactly does this mean? The DASH diet guidelines can help you understand exactly what to eat. Following these, alongside stopping smoking, becoming more active and drinking within the alcohol recommendations can help your systolic and diastolic blood pressure reduce.

As with most conditions, some people are more at risk of complications than others. In this case, men, older people and African Caribbean populations are all at higher risk of complications, making it even more important to make changes. The Premier study was a large study that followed more than 800 adults for 18 months. The participants were split into groups: Group A was given advice only, Group B had to follow a lifestyle change programme, and Group C followed the lifestyle change programme plus the DASH diet. The DASH diet group showed the biggest improvements in blood pressure. The study also showed that the greatest reductions in blood pressure were seen in people of African American descent and older people who had high blood pressure, so if you fall into either category, there is even more incentive to make changes.[2]

The DASH diet is a proven way to eat that will help people with high blood pressure and a risk of cardiovascular diseases. The research studies show us that it has the most significant impact on people who have high blood pressure to start with, or those with a higher BMI. Personally, I think this way of eating will benefit most of the population, so unless there are specific medical problems like those mentioned at the end of the chapter (see page 30), this way of eating should be healthy for your whole family.

Conditions where the DASH diet can help:

- If you have a family history of heart disease.
- If you have high blood pressure.
- If you have high cholesterol.
- If you have normal blood pressure but are concerned about your heart health.
- If you are overweight/obese.
- If you want an overall healthy, balanced way of eating for life.

The original DASH trial

With a steep increase in deaths from heart disease over the past 50 years, it became obvious that something needed to change. As healthcare professionals, we have to be led by the evidence, so back in the nineties, some large-scale research was done to look into this. The original research was carried out to see if diet alone would make a difference. They found that in anyone with high or normal blood pressure, diet changes were able to decrease systolic blood pressure by 6–11mmHg.[3] In 1992, the National Institute of Health (NIH) started some research comparing three different diets. More than 450 people over the age of 20, with stage 1 and 2 hypertension, took part.

The diets compared were:

- **a control diet** (similar to the normal Western diet – high in fat and salt, low in fruit and vegetables)
- **a diet higher in fruit and vegetables** (the normal Western diet, but with more fruit and vegetables)
- **the DASH diet**

Initially, everyone was asked to follow the control diet for three weeks. This was a test period to see who had sticking power and to get a baseline. Those who wanted to continue then kept eating the control diet or moved to eating either a diet with increased fruit and vegetables or the DASH diet for 8 weeks. All meals were provided, participants were told exactly what to eat and drink, and some meals were eaten on-site. This made it a very well-controlled research study.

The results were astounding. The DASH diet lowered systolic blood pressure by 5.5mmHg and diastolic by 3mmHg. The fruit and vegetable diet also lowered blood pressure, but not by as much (3mmHg systolic and 2mmHg diastolic).[4] People with type 1 hypertension saw their blood pressure decrease more significantly (by 11mmHg systolic and 5.5mmHg diastolic). These reductions were seen in just two weeks of making the dietary changes. It should be pointed out at this stage that 60 per cent of the people in this study were of African American descent, and we now know that this population group have a much higher risk of high blood pressure. This means people of African-American descent are at greater risk of heart disease, but also that they get greater benefits from the DASH diet.

It all sounds pretty good, doesn't it? It is. However, there are always limitations to be aware of. While the participants were provided with all the food they would eat to help them stick to the diet during the study, this isn't realistic for daily life. This book will give you recipes and the outline of what to eat, but it won't shop and cook for you! The participants in the study group were also provided with motivational sessions, education and support to keep them on track.[5] It's a lot easier to follow an eating plan when you have your food cooked for you, and someone motivating you, reminding you, checking on you and cheering you along, isn't it? This was highlighted by the fact that, after the study ended, despite all the significant health improvements seen, not many people stuck to the DASH diet. My hope is that this book will teach you how to eat for life, by helping you learn to plan your meals and cook delicious food that is balanced and will help reduce your blood pressure for a lot longer than a few weeks. You will need to be your own cheerleader, or find someone to do it alongside you and make these changes together.

Key nutrients in the DASH diet

So why is the DASH diet so effective? It makes total sense, really, that eating more fruit, vegetables and wholegrains will improve your health. The DASH diet takes this a step further by suggesting portion sizes for different foods. It is the combination and balance of nutrients that makes the difference. Let's take a closer look at some of the key nutrients at play.

Potassium

A key player in regulating blood pressure, there is substantial evidence showing that high levels of potassium are associated with lower blood pressure. One such study is the INTERSALT study, which followed over 10,000 people in 32 countries.[6] This study measured the amount of sodium in people's urine over 24 hours. It concluded that salt is very much associated with blood pressure – the higher the salt intake, the higher the blood pressure across adults of all ages, both men and women.

Looking at other cultures who do not eat a Western diet can also give us interesting information. For example, the Yanomami tribe in Brazil follow a mostly vegetarian diet with a high potassium to sodium (salt) ratio, and they have low blood pressure with no hypertension.[7] Of course, there can be other factors at play; for example, this population are also very active. However, the wealth of evidence we have suggests that even a small increase in your potassium intake can lower blood pressure.

Potassium allows the body to get rid of excess fluid and keeps blood vessels open so the blood can flow through, meaning the heart doesn't have to work as hard and blood pressure can stay lower. There is a clever balancing system between sodium and potassium. Potassium helps increase the amount of sodium you excrete so that the levels are not too high in the bloodstream. A diet high in potassium and low in sodium helps regulate our blood pressure.

Where do we get potassium from? Fruit, vegetables, potatoes, nuts and seeds are all good sources. Eating more fruit and veg and less salt is the way forward. From studies on other cultures in isolated rural locations, we see that diets high in fruit and veg lead to only 1 per cent of people getting hypertension.[8]

Calcium

Calcium is well known for its benefits on bone health and teeth. What you may not know is that a high intake of calcium from food is linked with lower blood pressure and a lowered risk of developing hypertension. The main source of calcium is dairy foods (milk, yogurt, cheese); however, it can also be found in lower quantities in other foods, such as green vegetables, tofu, bread, nuts and seeds.

The DASH diet recommends 3–4 servings of dairy a day to meet your calcium needs. If you do not consume cows' milk, you can still meet your calcium needs by ensuring your plant-based alternatives contain calcium.

Magnesium

We are less clear about magnesium's role with regard to blood pressure, but we know it is important. The DASH trial showed that when following the diet, participants had an increase in the amount of magnesium they were eating and excreting. Foods rich in magnesium include wholegrains, nuts and some fruit and vegetables.

Sodium

Too much sodium prevents the production of nitric oxide, a chemical that helps keep our arteries open so the blood can flow through easily.[9] Therefore, we want a diet that is higher in potassium than sodium – the recommended ratio is 5:1 (five times the amount of potassium to sodium).[10] This is not the case with the traditional Western diet. Ultra-processed convenience foods and salty snacks mean the average diet provides a ratio of 1:2 (twice the amount of sodium to potassium).

Because it is based on cooking from scratch using lean proteins, wholegrains, fruit and vegetables, the DASH diet is naturally lower in sodium. It aims for no more than 2,300mg sodium a day. There is also a lower salt version of the DASH diet, which aims for no more than 1,500mg sodium a day, and can give you additional reductions in blood pressure.

Key micronutrients for blood pressure

	Vegetables	Fruit
Potassium-rich foods	artichokes, asparagus, bamboo shoots, beetroot, broccoli, Brussels sprouts, butternut squash, carrots, cauliflower, celery, kale, mushrooms, okra, pumpkins, spinach, spring greens, sweet potatoes, tomatoes	apricots, avocados, bananas, cantaloupe melons, dried fruit (such as apples, apricots and dates, pears and peaches), grapefruit, honeydew melons, kiwi fruit, oranges, strawberries, tangerines
Calcium-rich foods	leafy green vegetables (such as kale, spinach and spring greens)	dried figs
Magnesium-rich foods	cassava, spinach, Swiss chard	avocados, bananas, figs, raisins

Nuts/seeds	Other
almonds, Brazil nuts, cashew nuts, chestnuts, hazelnuts, peanuts, pecans, pumpkin seeds, sunflower seeds, tofu, walnuts	beans, bran, coffee, molasses, muesli, potatoes, tea
almonds, chia seeds, poppy seeds, sesame seeds	cheese, cottage cheese, fromage frais, mackerel, milk, pilchards, salmon, canned sardines, soybeans (edamame beans), tahini, tofu, white beans, yogurt
almonds, Brazil nuts, cashew nuts, flaxseeds (linseeds), hazelnuts, macadamia nuts, peanuts, pecans, pistachios, pumpkin seeds, sesame seeds, sunflower seeds, walnuts	amaranth, barley, beans and lentils, bran, brown rice, buckwheat, bulgur wheat, granola, millet, plain dark chocolate, potatoes with skins, rolled oats, rye, soybeans (edamame beans), triticale, whole wheat, wild rice, tofu

Dietary fibre

Dietary fibre helps to slow the absorption of sugars, which is essential to the management of type 2 diabetes, weight management and overall health. Many of the benefits associated with fibre relate to bowel health, rendering it a not very sexy nutrient.

There are two types of fibre: insoluble and soluble. Insoluble fibre is the roughage that keeps our bowels regular, found in the skins of fruit and vegetables, the outer parts of wholegrains, and in seeds. It may also help to reduce the risk of colon cancer. Soluble fibre makes the stool softer, bulkier, more formed and thus easier to move through the colon. It can also help reduce cholesterol levels. It is found in oats, barley, fruit (apples, pears and oranges), beans, lentils and vegetables. All foods found in the DASH diet!

In the UK, it is recommended that you eat 30g fibre a day, but at the last count, the National Health and Diet Survey showed the average eaten was only about 20g a day. Eating 4–5 servings of fruit and 4–5 servings of vegetables each day will add plenty of fibre. Eating wholegrains will certainly boost your fibre intake, and by adding in some beans, pulses and nuts, you can easily reach the recommended 30g per day.

A word of warning: a rapid increase of fibre can cause bloating and gas, so it is a good idea to increase your intake in stages. Add an extra couple of portions of fruit and vegetables in the first week and then add the same again the following week. When you increase your fibre intake, you also need to increase your fluid, so make sure you drink plenty of water or you may end up constipated.

Omega-3 fatty acids

Omega-3s are known for being in oily (or smellier!) fish. They can reduce certain fats in the blood, reduce inflammation in the body and reduce your blood pressure, too. One study found taking 3g a day of omega-3s significantly decreased both systolic and diastolic blood pressure.[11] While this is all good news if you have high blood pressure, it is also something to be aware of for those who have low blood pressure. You can have too much of a good thing, so it is recommended we only eat 1–2 portions of oily fish a week.

Saturated fat

This is one that is reduced in the DASH diet. As you eat less confectionery, ultra-processed foods and red meat, and switch to reduced-fat dairy products, your saturated fat intake will fall. While our bodies need some saturated fat, too much can increase the risk of chronic diseases.

> **'If these nutrients are the key, then why can't I just take a supplement and keep my normal diet?'**
> When these nutrients have been tested individually, they have some impact on reducing blood pressure, but it is nowhere near the impact of following the DASH diet. There is something in the mix of these nutrients that is the key. When we eat nutrients in food, the body deals with them very differently to an individual supplement. One key difference is that the fibre in fruit and veg alters how we digest

food. Taking too much of one nutrient can mean that another nutrient cannot do its job, as there is competition between them. For example, taking too much of one B vitamin might flood the system so that another B vitamin cannot get in and work. Eating whole foods means the body can work this out rather than us prescribing what we think it needs.

Evidence base in other conditions

If you have high blood pressure, this may mean that you have other health issues. The good news is that the benefits of the DASH diet are not just for blood pressure. There have been improvements seen in so many health conditions, including type 2 diabetes and metabolic syndrome (see below), so by eating this way, you can improve your overall health.

Type 2 diabetes

In type 2 diabetes, the higher fibre content of the DASH diet can help with blood sugar control, preventing the large highs and lows. Wholegrains, fruit, vegetables, low-fat dairy and protein are all beneficial foods groups to be eating and can help with the control of type 2 diabetes. If you are concerned about the natural sugars present in fruit, then combining this with a protein or high-fibre food will help slow the rate at which the sugar is released into your bloodstream. Try eating fruit as part of a meal or combining it in a snack with a protein. For example, eat fruit with nuts, seeds, yogurt, hummus, nut butter, reduced-fat cheese, roasted chickpeas, cottage cheese or boiled eggs.

Metabolic syndrome

The DASH diet can also help in metabolic syndrome. Metabolic syndrome or Syndrome X is a combination of symptoms that puts you at greater risk of coronary heart disease and stroke.

Symptoms of metabolic syndrome include having more than three of the following:[12]

- waist circumference greater than 94cm (37 inches) for white, Black African, Middle Eastern and mixed origin men (above 90cm/35½ inches for South Asian, Asian and Black Caribbean men), and greater than 80cm (31½ inches) in all women.
- High levels of triglycerides and low HDL in the blood.
- Consistent blood pressure of 140/90mmHg or higher.
- Insulin resistance.
- An increased risk of developing blood clots (e.g. deep vein thrombosis).
- A tendency to develop irritation and swelling of the body tissue.

Insulin resistance is when the body does not respond well to the insulin it makes. This means that the blood sugars stay higher for longer than normal after you eat. The body will try to help by pumping out extra insulin, but this produces more cholesterol, and we end up storing the sugar in fat cells, where it is converted to fat. Over time, the body can stop producing enough insulin, resulting in type 2 diabetes.

Another side effect is that our liver tries to reduce the blood sugar level by converting it into another type of fat known as triglycerides, which increases the risk of heart disease. The good news is that the DASH diet can help with the majority of metabolic syndrome symptoms: it has shown improvements in insulin sensitivity, reductions in total cholesterol, improved glucose control and an overall reduction of stress in the body.[13] Ensure you focus on eating from the wholegrain food group, as wholegrains provide the fibre needed to help with blood sugar control.

Conditions to be more careful of

Extra guidance and advice should be taken with regards to the specific conditions listed below. The DASH diet can be helpful for these conditions, but it is a good idea to check with a dietitian or your healthcare team before starting on the DASH diet if you have any of the following:

- chronic kidney disease
- type 1 diabetes
- hypertension in pregnancy

Although the meals in this book are family meals, the DASH diet is not specifically designed for children. They have extra energy needs, and may need additional snacks on top of the meal plans in this book, as well as a slightly different balance of foods.

3
Getting Started on the DASH Diet

The DASH diet does not set out 'good' and 'bad' foods to either eat or eliminate from your diet. Instead, this is a way of eating where you focus on eating more plant-based and heart-healthy foods, and balancing these with those foods higher in fat, salt and sugar that our bodies need less often.

Instead of focusing on what *not* to eat, let's focus on what to eat more of, using servings as a guide. The number of servings you can eat will depend on how many calories your body needs. The calorie guide is in no way meant to encourage you to count calories, as that takes us into the realms of this being a diet where we count, restrict and feel guilty. It is just a guide to show how many servings of a food to aim for.

An average woman requires 2,000kcals a day and a man 2,500kcals a day. The 1,600kcals intake is aimed at women who are attempting to lose weight. Men who are trying to lose weight should follow the 2,000kcals plan. On pages 34–35 you will find a table giving you an idea for three different calorie intakes, and on page 85 you'll find guidance about which plan is right for you. If you are aiming to lose weight, standard advice is to reduce your calorie intake by 500kcals but bear in mind that you are also aiming to be more active and change the types of foods you eat. Unless you have been tracking how many calories you eat, you also won't know your starting point. The best way to know how much to eat is to start to tune into your internal body cues. Think about what hunger feels like in your body, what thirst feels like and what fullness feels like. Setting your calorie intake too low may just lead to hunger, leading you to fill up on high-fat and sugary foods that feel satisfying. If this is happening regularly, then please do add in an extra snack a day with fruit or vegetables and protein. Tracking your hunger levels over a few days can highlight where those hungry points of the day are. Instead of ignoring hunger, can you have your next meal a little earlier or respond with a suitable snack? An apple with almonds or carrot sticks with hummus can keep you satisfied until your next meal.

Start with the calories suggested for your gender. Keep a food diary for a week and then count up the servings of the food groups that you already consume. In the beginning, you may feel quite overwhelmed by the target. Do not panic! This is a way of eating for life, therefore you do not need to make instant changes overnight. Take it slowly. If you cannot meet the number of servings straight away, you could instead decide to focus on one food group at a time, or increase your servings every few weeks as you adapt to this new way of eating. There is no right or wrong way to do this.

Here is an example. Dave is an office worker who doesn't have a very active lifestyle. He has recently been diagnosed with high blood pressure and wants to try altering his lifestyle before using medications. He is going to start on the 2,500kcal meal plan and increase his activity. He plans to do 30 minutes of exercise daily by walking to work and then having one longer walk at the weekend. Dave considers his food intake for a week. This table shows his food intake on an average weekday:

Breakfast	Honey hoops with semi-skimmed milk and a banana
Snack	Chocolate bar
Lunch	Wholemeal sandwich with ham and cheese, apple, crisps
Dinner	White pasta with tomato sauce, chicken, peas and mushrooms
Snack	Salted nuts

Dave notes that his current daily intake is two portions of vegetables, two portions of fruit, two servings of wholegrain foods, one portion of dairy, two portions of lean meat and some nuts – but these are salted. Some initial changes he makes include switching to a wholegrain cereal and pasta, adding raw vegetables and a glass of fruit juice to his lunch, and having a yogurt and fruit topped with unsalted nuts for an evening snack. This feels achievable and brings him to three portions of vegetables, four of fruit and two of dairy, plus six wholegrain foods and two lean meats a day. He isn't yet meeting his targets, but it's a great start that he can then build on, making further changes in a few weeks' time and increasing his fruit and vegetables further.

Here are the more specific portion guides for using calories as a guide:[1]

Food group	1,600kcals	2,000kcals
Wholegrain foods	6 servings per day	6-8 servings per day
Vegetables	3-4 servings per day	4-5 servings per day
Fruit	4 servings per day	4-5 servings per day
Dairy	2-3 servings per day	3 servings per day
Lean proteins	3-6 servings per day	Up to 6 servings per day
Nuts, seeds	3 servings per week	4-5 servings per week
Fats and oils	2 servings per day	2-3 servings per day
Sugars	Up to 3 servings per week	Up to 5 servings per week

	2,500kcals	One serving
	10–11 servings per day	1 slice of wholegrain/rye bread, ½ medium pitta, ½ large wholemeal wrap, 3 wholemeal oatcakes/crackers, 30g (1oz) dry wholegrain cereal, 25g (⅘oz) rolled oats, 30g (1oz) uncooked wholegrain (brown) rice, 25g (⅘oz) uncooked wholewheat pasta or other wholegrains
	5–6 servings per day	1 large cupped handful (80g/2¾oz) cooked or raw veg, 2 handfuls (120g/4¼oz) leafy greens
	4–5 servings per day	1 handful (80g/2¾oz)
	3 servings per day	200ml (⅓ pint) semi-skimmed or skimmed milk, 4 tablespoons (150g/5½oz) low-fat yogurt, 45g (1¾oz) Cheddar cheese (or similar hard cheese – reduced fat if you choose)
	Up to 6 servings per day	1 egg, 25g (⅘oz) lean meat/fish (cooked weight), 125g (4½oz) beans or pulses
	1 serving per day	50g (1¾oz) nuts, 2 tablespoons (40g/1½oz) nut butter, 2 tablespoons (16–30g/½–1oz) seeds
	3 servings per day	1 teaspoon reduced-fat olive oil spread or vegetable oil, 1 tablespoon low-fat mayo, 1 tablespoon normal salad dressing or 2 tablespoons low-fat salad dressing
	Up to 5 servings per week	1 tablespoon sugar, jam or jelly, 1 glass of lemonade, 125g (4½oz) sorbet, ice cream or frozen yogurt, 1 fancy biscuit, 2 plain biscuits, 1 slice of plain cake, ½ slice of fancier cake

Please do note, I am not advocating that you track your calories each day, as that is unrealistic and feeds into diet culture. Instead, this is about focusing on servings so that, in time, you can find a balanced and sustainable way of eating. Remember the original DASH study, where people were not able to stick to the plan after the research ended? It isn't always easy to make a large change to your eating all in one go, so try setting smaller goals and gradually building up. I recommend you keep a journal to track what you're currently eating (see pages 38–9 for a template you can use). Complete this table for three days and then find the average number of portions in each food group. You can also create a goal-setting chart (see page 40 for a template) so you can see how many changes there are to make. Maybe you could start by increasing your fruit and vegetables by a couple of portions a day for two weeks, and then try switching to more wholegrain foods. Building up slowly in this way can also help your body adjust to the increase in fibre. As mentioned earlier, when you increase your fibre intake, you want to do it slowly, as it can lead to pain or discomfort and bloating in some people. Also, remember to keep up with your fluid intake to help prevent constipation. When you have achieved your first couple of goals, plan the next changes. This could be switching your dairy to lower-fat options and eating nuts three times a week as a snack. Remember, this is a lifelong approach and it can seem quite overwhelming at first. Planning it out in manageable steps will help make it feel more achievable.

How to start – cupboards and meal-planning

If you have tasty, easy-to-access food at home, you are more likely to eat it. A supply of fresh, frozen, dried and canned foods will give you plenty of options. To help you get started, this book has a 21-day meal plan with a shopping list for each week (see chapter 7). Hopefully, once you've used it a few times, you will be in the swing of the DASH lifestyle and have a few other recipes you can add to your repertoire.

Every time you find a good recipe, I recommend you write it out and pop it in a folder, whether that is a saved folder on your phone or a real one! Social media can be a great place to find new recipe ideas, and if they are not quite DASH-friendly, you can adapt them: add extra vegetables, switch the grains and pop a salad on the side. On one day of the week you can sit down with your folder and recipe books, plus your diary. While it is important to make time to prepare food, you also need to plan around your week. On busier days, you will need super-quick meals or to reheat a portion made on another day. When you have more time, batch-cooking is your friend, or might decide to cook a more extravagant meal that takes more effort and time.

When you meal-plan, I'd advise you start out planning for all three meals per day and for snacks too. This may feel like it's OTT, but it will help you stay on track to meet your DASH portions and enable you to feel like you know what you are doing! As a general guide, you need your three main meals to each contain two portions of wholegrain foods, one or two portions of vegetables and one portion of fruit, plus two portions of protein and a dairy portion, either with the meal or as a dessert. The rest you can then have as snacks.

My current day's food:

What I currently eat	Wholegrain foods	Fruit	Veggies	Dairy
Breakfast				
Snack				
Lunch				
Snack				
Dinner				
Dessert				
Snack				

Lean proteins	Nuts, seeds, beans and pulses	Fats and oils	Sugars

Goal-setting chart:

	How many portions I currently eat	Goal 1	Goal 2	Goal 3	DASH Goal
Wholegrain foods					
Fruit					
Veggies					
Dairy					
Lean proteins					
Nuts, seeds, beans and pulses					
Fats and oils					
Sugars					

Some examples of small changes you can make as you work towards your DASH goals:

	Original food intake	Portions	Changes made	Portions
Breakfast	Non-wholegrain cereal with milk	1 dairy	Oats with fruit, milk and a sprinkle of seeds	2 wholegrain 1 fruit 1 dairy 1 seeds
Snack	Fruit	1 fruit	Fruit	1 fruit
Lunch	Sandwich (sometimes wholemeal and sometimes white bread) using butter with tuna mayo and cucumber	0–2 wholegrain 1 veggies 2 protein 1 fat	Wholemeal sandwich with olive oil spread, tuna with reduced-fat mayo, salad and chopped raw veggies on the side	2 wholegrain 2 veggies 2 protein 1 fat
Snack	Cake and fruit	1 sugar 1 fruit	Popcorn and Cheddar cheese (reduced fat, if you choose)	1 wholegrain 1 dairy
Dinner	Spaghetti Bolognese (non wholemeal pasta) with 1 portion of veggies. Cooking with olive oil	1 veggie 1 oil 2 protein	Spaghetti Bolognese with wholemeal pasta, 2 portions of veggies and a side salad	2 wholegrain 3 veggies 2 protein
Dessert	Fizzy drink and chocolate	1 fat 1 sugar	Yogurt with fruit and dark chocolate, and sparkling water	1 dairy 1 fruit 1 sugar
Snack	Biscuits	1 sugar	Nuts and fruit	1 nuts 1 fruit
Total portions		0–2 wholegrain 4 fruit 2 veggies 1 dairy 4 protein 2 fat 2 sugar		7 wholegrain 4 fruit 5 veggies 4 dairy 3 protein 2 nuts and seeds 1 fat 1 sugar

	How many portions I currently eat a day	Goal 1
Wholegrain foods	1	Switch to wholemeal bread and oats for breakfast 4
Fruit	2	Add fruit to breakfast daily 3
Veggies	2	Add a side salad to dinner 3
Dairy	1	Have yogurt for dessert 2
Lean proteins	6	
Nuts, seeds, beans and pulses per week	0	Add nuts to lunch/ as a snack 4–5 times a week
Fats and oils	4	Switch from butter to reduced-fat olive oil spread and low-fat mayo 3
Sugars	21–28 per week	Switch from fizzy drinks to sparkling water 14

Goal 2	Goal 3	DASH Goal
Add popcorn or oatcakes as a snack 5	Switch to wholegrain (brown) rice, whole-wheat pasta or other wholegrain foods at dinner 6-7	6-8
Have two pieces of fruit as a snack or with yogurt for dessert 5		4-5
Have chopped veggies as a snack or with lunch 4		4-5
Add yogurt to your oats for breakfast 3		3
		Up to 6
		4-5
		2-3
Switch from biscuits as a snack to oatcakes or popcorn 7	Reduce cake intake to once a week 5	Up to 5 per week

Example of how you may want to spread out the portions of food:

	1,600kcals	2,000kcals	2,500kcals
Breakfast	2 x wholegrain foods 1 x fruit 1 x dairy	2 x wholegrain foods 1 x fruit 1 x dairy	3 x wholegrain foods 1 x fruit 1 x dairy
Lunch	2 x wholegrain foods 1 x fruit 2 x veggies 2 x lean proteins	2 x wholegrain foods 1 x fruit 2 x veggies 2 x lean proteins	3 x wholegrain foods 1 x fruit 2 x veggies 3 x lean proteins
Dinner	2 x wholegrain foods 2 x veggies 2 x lean proteins	2 x wholegrain foods 3 x veggies 3 x lean proteins	3 x wholegrain foods 3 x veggies 3 x lean proteins
Dessert	1 x dairy 1 x fruit	1 x dairy 1 x fruit	1 x dairy 2 x fruit 1 x nuts
Snacks	1 x fruit Nuts on some days Up to 3 sweet foods a week	1 x wholegrain food 1 x fruit Up to 5 sweet foods a week	1 x wholegrain food 1 x dairy 1 x veggies 1 x fruit Up to 5 sweet foods a week

Fresh fruit and vegetables can be lovely to snack on and grab right from the fruit bowl, but will not keep for long, so you will need to shop weekly and then keep a close eye on what needs using up first. I'd recommend making friends with your local greengrocer, as they are likely to be the cheapest supplier for your fresh food and will often have deals or a box of reduced goods that need eating quickly before they go off. This can keep your costs down. Or look into having a fruit and vegetable box delivered; this can be a little more expensive, but will often contain locally grown produce and minimal plastic, so you're helping the environment too.

By the end of the week, if your fresh produce has all been used up, plan to use frozen and canned produce. Frozen fruit and vegetables can be a real timesaver, as having them ready chopped and peeled makes them so easy to cook with, and they can stay in the freezer for several months. Plus you can buy things that are hard to keep fresh (such as berries) or tricky to buy good-quality versions of locally (such as mangos or soybeans/edamame beans).

I love to keep a supply of frozen vegetables, as it means I always have plenty of veggies available. Buying vegetables like butternut squash and onions frozen can be useful if you don't like preparing them, or if you only use them in small quantities. Reseal with a clip and they will keep for a long time.

Let's not forget about canned foods. Stock up on canned beans, lentils and vegetables – all in water with low/no sugar and salt. And, of course, the humble canned tomatoes, used in so many meals! A selection of cans can make a super-fast meal – chopped tomatoes combined with canned beans, peas and sweetcorn, along with some spices, makes you a tasty bean chilli! Other great canned foods to keep in your cupboard include coconut milk, potatoes, tuna and other fish. Canned fruit can make a yummy dessert – go for options in juice, not syrup.

Make sure you have a supply of your favourite spices, herbs and condiments, as these make all the difference to cooking tasty meals. Low-salt stock cubes, dried chilli flakes, ground cumin and coriander (or whole seeds you can crush yourself) and dried mixed herbs are some of my essentials. Balsamic vinegar, low-salt soy sauce, fish sauce, peanut butter, low-fat mayonnaise, olive oil and a range of other vinegars are also key ingredients to have on hand.

Keep fresh garlic in your kitchen and fresh ginger in your freezer – you can grate this from frozen, skin and all. Growing some fresh herbs will add that flourish to a meal. It's very easy to grow your own thyme, rosemary and sage, so pop to the garden centre and pick up a few nice herbs while you are planning.

Have bag clips, wax wraps or resealable, reusable bags ready to store leftovers and fresh produce in the refrigerator. If you store snack food pre-chopped, it can help you snack on the right things. Or you could buy it already chopped – a little more expensive, but worth it if it means you eat it.

If you work away from home, stock up on dried fruit, nuts, seeds, wholegrain crackers and wholegrain breadsticks for your desk drawer, or plan to take healthy snacks in with you daily. Good office snacks include individual cheese portions with wholegrain crackers and grapes, carrot sticks and hummus (take in a pile for a few weeks/snacks), individual pots of yogurt and pots of fruit in natural juice. Use a mini insulated bag with a freezer block if you do not have access to a refrigerator. It is useful to always have more than you think you need! Bring in extra supplies for those days that you cannot get to a shop, and always keep a snack in your bag for those moments you get caught out when out and about.

Planning is really key here. You do not want to skip meals or snacks, as this leads to hunger, which may lead to you overeating other foods. Instead, plan out your week, think about where you will be and whether you need food with you, and have a reserve snack 'just in case'.

4

Key Food Groups

Each of the food groups included in the DASH diet are there for a specific reason. Of course, individual nutrients are important in their own right, but it is actually the *combination* of these nutrients in the food groups that brings the benefits and makes nutrition so fascinating. In this section, we will look in depth at each group, the foods that are in it and the nutritional science.

Wholegrains

Wholegrains are the seeds of cereal plants. They include: brown rice, wild rice, amaranth, bulgur wheat, maize, corn, quinoa, couscous, oats, millet, rye, buckwheat, freekeh, barley, pumpernickel and sorghum. Wholegrains are the whole versions of grains and they have three layers: bran, germ and endosperm. Each part contains slightly different nutrients:

- The **endosperm** is in the centre and provides starch.
- The **germ** provides protein, healthy fats, B vitamins and vitamin E.

- The **bran** is the outer layer. It provides B vitamins, insoluble fibre (the type needed by your gut bacteria) and phytochemicals.

Refined grains are the white versions of carbohydrate foods, like white rice, flour, pasta, white bread, pastries, cakes and biscuits. They have the bran and germ removed, which takes away a lot of the nutrients and makes them lower in fibre – and often lower in mineral content too.

Because wholegrains contain all three layers of the grain, they give you all those B vitamins, fibre and nutrients. Rolled, crushed and cracked versions all count (e.g. cracked bulgur wheat, rolled oats). They are also low in saturated fat and salt. For a food to be called wholegrain, there must be at least 51 per cent of a wholegrain ingredient present by weight. Be aware that just because a food is brown, it doesn't mean it's wholegrain! Another trick used by the food industry is to use caramel/brown food colouring, which is slightly misleading, so do check out the nutrition label for the amount of wholegrain in a food. Look out for foods labelled as 100 per cent wholegrain or wholewheat, or look to see where wholegrains are in the ingredients list. The higher up the list, the more wholegrains in the food.

Why eat wholegrains?

Wholegrains have definite heart health benefits and can lower the risk of heart disease. A review of 10 studies showed eating 3 x 28g (1oz) servings a day may lower your risk of heart disease by 22 per cent, and the benefits continued with eating up to seven portions of wholegrains a day.[1] They may also help with weight management, as their high fibre content makes them filling. Being plant compounds, wholegrains contain plenty of micronutrients, including polyphenols, stanols and sterols, which can help lower cholesterol and have benefits for our heart health.

Wholegrains are classified as low in glycemic index, which means they do not cause as large an increase in blood sugar as the white, refined alternatives. All carbohydrates are broken down into glucose: the difference is that the fibre in wholegrains slows down the impact on blood sugars. You can see how this would be beneficial if you have type 2 diabetes or metabolic syndrome. It can also help with weight reduction, as having better control of your blood sugars can help keep you fuller for longer. Making simple switches over to wholemeal, wholegrain, wholewheat (pasta) or brown options is a great move to help your heart.

With the portions in the DASH diet, you may need to have more than one portion of wholegrain foods per meal. You may have two or three portions at each meal: two slices of toast at breakfast, one large wrap for lunch and a cup of cooked grains in the evening comes to six portions in the day. This does not mean you have free passage to eat large portions of grains. It is very easy to overeat carbohydrate foods, and this can be one reason that people struggle with their weight. While I wouldn't recommend you get into the habit of weighing your carbs out daily, it can be a useful thing to do right at the start of this process to give you an idea of what a portion should be. Try weighing out your normal portion, then weigh out a DASH portion and compare it. Then, a top tip is to create your own measuring device: I like using cups or a specific serving ladle. You can mark out where the different grains come to on your measuring device, and then there is no need to weigh it each time. Knowing how much rice, pasta and other grains to cook means sensible portion sizes – and also no waste!

Fats and oils

Years ago, it was all the rage to eat a low-fat diet. We now know that the science on this was not quite correct. You do not need to eat a low-fat diet, but you do want to be conscious of what types of fats you are eating.

The main types of fat are saturated and unsaturated – these terms are derived from the amount of hydrogen atoms attached to the fatty acids that make up the fat. If a fatty acid is holding the maximum number of hydrogen atoms, it is saturated, whereas if there are hydrogen atoms missing in the chain, the fat is unsaturated. There are also different types of unsaturated fat, depending on the structure of the fat cell.

Saturated fats are holding the maximum number of hydrogen atoms. These tend to come from animal fats – think of the white fat on a piece of meat, or butter, cheese and lard – and also include coconut oil. They are solid at room temperature. Eat less of these for your heart health.

Unsaturated fats can either be **monounsaturated** – missing hydrogen in one spot (mono = one) – or **polyunsaturated** – missing more than two hydrogen atoms (poly = many). Both types are liquid at room temperature.

Monounsaturated fats are heart-healthy, as are small amounts of polyunsaturated fats. Monounsaturates include olive oil, rapeseed oil, avocados and certain nuts. Eating more of these and fewer saturated fats can help lower your cholesterol and risk of heart disease. These fats may also reduce inflammation in the body and have been shown to aid weight loss.

The two main types of polyunsaturated fats are omega-3s and omega-6s, which you may have heard of already. Omega-3s provide alpha-linolenic acid (ALA), an essential fatty acid that you need to have in your diet. ALA is converted into two other fatty acids, DHA (docosahexaenoic acid) and EPA (eicosapentaenoic acid). The omega-3 fatty acids are a fascinating type of fat. They can help lower your blood pressure, reduce inflammation in the body and increase levels of the beneficial HDL cholesterol. The best sources are oily fish (trout, salmon, herring, kippers, fresh tuna, sardines, mackerel) as they contain EPA and DHA in their pure form. Plant sources of omega-3s have to be converted to EPA and DHA – this process means they are not as effective as oily fish, but they are still highly nutritious DASH foods. Examples are tahini, chia seeds, flaxseeds (linseeds), walnuts and pine nuts.

Trans fats (also known as hydrogenated fats) are man-made fats that are sometimes found in cakes, biscuits and snack foods. You can look for these fats on food labels – check for the word 'hydrogenated'. These fats are being reduced in our food, so hopefully you won't find too many of them!

By following the portion advice in this book, you should find that the fat content of your diet becomes better for your heart. For heart health reasons, you want to eat less saturated fat and trans fat, but rather than reduce these and eat more of just any food group, you specifically want to eat more monounsaturated and polyunsaturated fats. It is a case of swapping fats, rather than not eating any fat at all.

Some simple fat swaps you can make are to switch to using rapeseed or olive oil for cooking, to use an olive oil-based reduced-fat spread instead of butter, and to use reduced-fat cheese. Eating oily fish once or twice a week and adding nuts and seeds to your diet will help with that all-important omega-3 intake. Choose olive oil, rapeseed oil, olives, avocados, almonds, cashew nuts, 100 per cent nut butters and sesame seeds.

Fat and cholesterol

Cholesterol is made from fat and protein, and high levels of it is associated with heart disease. The DASH diet can also lower cholesterol – back in the original research, it lowered total cholesterol by 13.7mg/dL, with a bigger decrease in the LDL compared to the HDL.[2] This is what we want to see! We talked about what cholesterol is earlier in the book (see page 12), now let's talk about how the DASH diet can help.

If your cholesterol is high, then you may have heard of plant stanols/sterols. These have a similar structure to cholesterol and act to reduce the amount of cholesterol absorbed in the body. If less cholesterol is absorbed, your cholesterol levels reduce. There are a variety of margarines/ fat spreads and yogurts containing these plant compounds. You can use these as part of the DASH diet if you want to, but it may not be necessary, as you will be naturally increasing your fruit, vegetable and wholegrain consumption. This means you will consume more sterols/stanols naturally. This, combined with regular exercise and a balanced diet, should help your cholesterol without the need for more expensive food items.

Fruit and vegetables

In 2017, the Global Burden of Disease study found that a diet low in fruit was the third biggest dietary risk factor for death from a chronic disease such as obesity, cancer and CVD.[3] So all fruit can be considered a super food! You can see why, as fruit provides fibre, potassium, magnesium, some calcium and plenty of vitamin C. There are also plenty of micronutrients in there that act as antioxidants, fighting disease in the body, or as probiotics, aiding our gut health.

The DASH diet recommends you eat 8–10 portions of fruit and vegetables a day (that's 4–5 portions of fruit and 4–5 portions of veg). This may sound like a lot and, quite frankly, it is when you compare it to the UK's average of four portions a day.[4]

So, where do you start? Look at what you currently eat: are there any meals without any fruit and vegetables in them at all? If so, begin there. Aim for 1–2 portions of fruit or vegetables with each meal and then eat the rest as snacks. You could have a breakfast of porridge with berries and a banana, a lunch with salad vegetables and some fruit, and a dinner with two vegetable portions. You can add in snacks of an apple and some carrot sticks.

Some vegetables don't count, but can catch you out: yams, potatoes, cassava and plantain count as starchy foods, not vegetables. Yes, I know they are vegetables when you grow and classify them, but nutritionally, they differ. Things that do count are fresh, frozen or canned fruit and vegetables (if canned, opt for natural juice or low-salt/sugar varieties). Dried fruit and fruit juices or smoothies can count only once a day. This is due to the levels of natural sugars in them, which is discussed below. Aim for as many colours of fruit and veggies as you can, as this helps you to get a variety of micronutrients and phytochemicals that fight disease and provide protection for the body.

'Isn't fruit full of sugar?'

Fruit contains natural sugars, but these do not have the same effect on health as eating free sugars in foods such as sweets, cakes, biscuits, soft drinks and desserts. Instead of reducing your fruit intake, you want to be increasing it! The sugar in fruit is pre-packaged in a matrix full of fibre, which means it is harder to get to, takes longer to digest and has a different effect on the body to eating a teaspoon of honey, for example. Fruit also contains all kinds of other nutrients that can be so beneficial to the body: vitamin C and potassium, to name a couple. There are so many phytochemicals and antioxidants in fruit that help the body fight disease and keep it healthy – nature knew what it was doing. For example, apples and pears contain carotenoids that have been shown to lower the risk of CVD. Berries contain flavonoids and anthocyanins that can help reduce LDL cholesterol levels and blood pressure, while increasing HDL cholesterol.

What counts as a portion?

A portion of fruit or vegetables is 80g (2¾oz). This is one medium-sized piece of fruit, two smaller pieces of fruit, 3 tablespoons vegetables or a dessert bowl of salad. A nice way to think about it is a portion being what fits into a cupped hand or a large handful of leafy vegetables.

A few special considerations

Dried fruit contains high levels of sugar that can stick to teeth, leading to tooth decay, so it is best to keep it to after mealtimes or as a part of a meal rather than as a snack. Fruit juice and smoothies have been contentious over the years. They can be a good way to get an extra portion of fruit and vegetables into your diet, but again, they contain higher levels of natural sugar. This also means that 150ml (¼ pint) juice only counts as one portion a day. No matter how many portions of fruit and vegetables you juice, it doesn't change this! Having your juice or smoothie with a meal will help prevent large spikes in blood sugars. If you are buying juices, stick to 100 per cent fruit juice that is unsweetened. Smoothies contain the whole fruit, and so they have more fibre. This means they do not have such a dramatic impact on blood sugar levels, but the sugar they contain is still more accessible to the body compared to eating the whole fruit.

Ways to eat more fruit and veg:

- Have fruit with your breakfast. For example, berries or a banana on your cereal, or an apple on the side.
- Always have two portions of vegetables with dinner. This may mean you need to add extra vegetables into your normal meals. Frozen vegetables work well in casseroles and stews, and you can add veg on the side or incorporate them into rice and pasta meals.
- Use beans or pulses in your cooking. This will reduce your meat and increase your vegetables. A handful of lentils can go into most meals.
- Add dried fruit at the end of the meal for that sweet hit, and to add an extra portion of fruit.
- Include fruit or vegetables as a snack and plan this so you have them accessible and ready. You can keep peeled sliced carrots and peppers in sealed bags in the refrigerator, or have sugar snap peas and mini cucumbers ready to munch.
- Don't forget: a juice or smoothie can only count once a day – and make sure you have it with a meal.
- Fruit served with yogurt and nuts is always a great dessert, or you can use fruit such as apples, pears or blackberries to bake a wholemeal crumble.
- Add a side salad to lunch. Salads can be so much more than lettuce, tomato and cucumber! Make them exciting and colourful, adding items like red cabbage, grated carrot, chopped broccoli and cauliflower, roasted aubergine and sweet potato, baby corn, sugar snap peas, soybeans (edamame beans), olives, gherkins and pickled onions. Sprouted seeds and

micro-greens such as pea shoots are also super tasty. You can grow these on a windowsill at home. A top tip is to keep pots of prepped salad ingredients in your refrigerator and then make your own salad bar.

- Grow your own varieties of salad leaves – baby spinach, rocket and mixed salad leaves are quick to grow on a windowsill or in pots. You could try out different versions of vegetables, like purple beans, yellow courgettes or round carrots. Items fresh from the ground can taste so much better, and it brings some real variety to your meals.

- Add extra veggies to your diet by roasting a tray of vegetables (courgettes, aubergines, peppers, tomatoes) and making your own pasta sauce, pizza sauce or Bolognese sauce. Roasted vegetables can be used in so many ways. They make a lovely addition to salads, or a perfect side dish to a meal that needs an extra portion of veggies.

- Get inventive with your sandwiches by adding in grated carrot, radishes for a peppery punch, micro-greens or sweetcorn.

- If there are vegetables you are not keen on, try them cooked in other ways. Raw vegetables can sometimes be overlooked – you can eat Brussels sprouts, broccoli and cauliflower raw. Try out the Cheesy Courgette Fingers recipe (see page 150) for a tasty way of trying out new veg, or why not whizz those vegetables into a soup? Over time, your palate will adapt and you will learn to really enjoy the freshness of the veg.

Here are some examples of what counts as a portion for different fruit and vegetables:

Fruit	Vegetables
1 apple/banana/pear	3 tablespoons sweetcorn/peas/carrots/frozen mixed veg
7 strawberries	4 heaped tablespoons leafy greens
2 satsumas/kiwi fruit/plums	a handful of broccoli spears/cauliflower florets
a large handful of berries or grapes	80g (2¾oz) beans/pulses (only counts once a day)
½ grapefruit or avocado	1 dessertbowl of salad
7 cherry tomatoes/2 tomatoes	
30g (1oz) dried fruit (1 tablespoon raisins)	
150ml (¼ pint) fruit juice or smoothie, unsweetened and 100 per cent juice (only once a day)	

An example of how to get your 10 portions a day:

- Porridge with banana and 1 tablespoon raisins (2)
- Snack of apple and nuts (1)
- Tuna sandwich with a side salad, plus 2 satsumas (2)
- Carrot sticks and hummus (1)
- Spaghetti Bolognese made with ½ meat, ½ lentils and two portions of vegetables (3)
- Yogurt and berries (1)

Dairy

Dairy foods include the following: yogurt, butter, cream, cheese, fromage frais, cream cheese, quark, milk and dairy calcium-fortified alternatives.

Now, you may be thinking, 'Hold on a minute, dairy is an animal product and high in saturated fat' – and you would be correct. Now and again, we get scare stories about dairy, one big one being that dairy causes high blood pressure. This comes from the Cornell China Study, which compared health data from rural China over a decade and found a strong link between milk intake and high blood pressure. However, as is often the case with research, we need to drill down deeper. This study looked at people in 65 areas in China. When you look, 62 of the 65 areas did not actually eat dairy at all, and the three areas that did were very different in terms of climate, lifestyle and eating. There are also questions over whether it was pasteurized milk being drunk or yaks' milk, which are very different. So there could have been many other factors at play. The consensus in the scientific research is that there is no strong link between dairy products and heart disease.[5]

What we do know is that dairy foods contain a fabulous range of nutrients that are good for general health. Dairy provides good-quality protein (for growth and repair of muscles), calcium (for bones, the nervous system and teeth), iodine (for the nervous system and brain), plus B vitamins (for energy release) and fat-soluble vitamins A, D, E and K. Eating three portions a day of these foods can help look after your bone health, so the DASH diet could help prevent osteoporosis and loss of bone density.[6]

Low-fat or full-fat dairy?

The original data on the DASH diet was based on low-fat dairy. Switching to low-fat dairy can reduce your calorie intake, so may be beneficial for weight loss. Indeed, for years, it was believed that eating a low-fat diet would aid weight loss, whereas we know now that our bodies need a certain level of fat, and that eating a very low-fat diet can lead to you craving other foods or missing out on certain nutrients.

Whereas full-fat dairy provides a whole host of vitamins and nutrients (see above), some lower fat versions are not as nutritious, containing higher levels of sugar and leaving you feeling unsatisfied. Therefore, I think this comes down to personal choice and common sense.

Milk is a fairly simple choice – go for semi-skimmed or skimmed milk for adults, and full-fat milk for infants and toddlers. Cheese is a little more complicated, as there are so many types. Milk has a saturated fat content of 2–3 per cent compared to cheese, which can contain up to 40 per cent. Cheeses such as Cheddar, double Gloucester, red Leicester, Brie and Stilton are high in fat at 20–40g of fat per 100g. Test out reduced-fat versions – these tend to contain 10–16g of fat per 100g, so can make quite a difference if you like them. Cottage cheese, quark and low-fat cream cheese are all good options to have on a more regular basis and mean you can then save the higher fat cheeses to savour and enjoy.

Yogurts are variable in taste and texture. A low-fat natural or Greek yogurt is a good choice, but if you really love the full-fat version, just go easy on the portion size. It is worth choosing a reduced-fat olive oil spread instead of butter, as butter is very high in saturated fat, which we know is linked to your cholesterol levels. It is worth trying the lower fat alternatives for a couple of weeks and seeing how you get on with them. If you are really not enjoying them, then perhaps you need a mix. If you don't like reduced-fat Cheddar cheese in a sandwich, but find it is fine grated on top of food, then buy a small amount of both. If low-fat yogurt is fine in a smoothie or baking, then go with that, but if you prefer full-fat yogurt when eating it with fruit, just be portion-aware.

Top tips: You can buy individual portions of cheeses for work or when you're out and about. Try mini portions, reduced-fat soft cheese in individual pots, or cut up reduced-fat hard cheese (like Cheddar) into portions yourself in advance. You can buy single serving pots of yogurts or use a glass jar to portion out yogurt from a large pot – this will also help you reduce the amount of plastic you use.

If you are lactose-intolerant, do not panic! The lactose in Greek yogurt is low and so you may well be able to tolerate it. Many hard cheeses are also low in lactose. Try reduced-fat Cheddar and see if it works for your body. Lactose-free milk is made from normal cows' milk, so already contains calcium. If you drink a plant-based milk, then it is important to check the label to ensure it is unsweetened and fortified with calcium – and preferably iodine and vitamin D too.

Lean protein sources

Your body is made up of about 20 per cent protein, and it should make up 15–35 per cent of your calories each day. Proteins are used to build muscles, tissues and organs; they also make up hormones and enzymes that help reactions occur in the body and are needed to digest food. Some proteins transport nutrients around the body, while others are involved in our immune system, keeping us healthy. Protein is also key for keeping us full up and helping to stabilize our blood sugars. You can see how important it is that we eat enough of it.

Where do we find protein?

Protein can be found in more foods than you probably realize. There is a small amount of protein in grains (pasta, oats, rice), but the main protein-rich foods are nuts, seeds, beans, dairy, meat, fish, soya, tofu and eggs.

There are so many protein foods you could be eating, so which ones are the best?

Protein is made up of building blocks known as amino acids. Nine of these amino acids are essential, which means they cannot be made by the body, but are needed for it to function properly. Others are non-essential, meaning the body is able to make them from other components. This is important when we think about the difference between animal and plant proteins. Animal proteins are known as complete proteins, as they contain the nine essential amino acids. Plant proteins usually lack at least one of the essential amino acids.

Does this mean we should eat meat over beans, pulses and other plant proteins?

I'd say as a general trend, we should be trying to increase the plant proteins that we eat. There is nothing wrong with eating meat: in fact, it is highly nutritious and can be an important source of nutrients such as iron, vitamin B12, vitamin D and zinc. However, it all comes down to balance. We don't need to be eating meat every day, especially red meat. Some research suggests that if you replace red meat once a day with another type of protein (poultry, fish or plant), then you could lower your risk of stroke by up to 27 per cent.[7] So, if you are a ham sandwich kind of person, try varying those lunch fillers with hummus, egg or tuna. There are plenty of ideas in the recipe section of this book (see chapter 6).

Is meat bad for our health?

A while ago, there was a lot of media coverage on red meat, and you may remember there being some scary headlines linking red meat with cancer. While there is some truth here, the research was observational, which means a group of people were observed over time. So this isn't a case of X definitely leads to Y, but rather a trend that the researchers noted, where people eating red meat appeared to be more likely to die from cancer.[8]

One of the key points to be aware of here is that the association seen was stronger with processed red meat (bacon, ham, sausages, salami) and with large portions of red meat – we are talking over 160g (5¾oz) per day. A normal portion of red meat should be around 70g (2½oz), so while 160g (5¾oz) may seem like a lot, if you had minced beef for dinner and a ham sandwich for lunch, you could easily be there.

Eating too much of any food group can be bad for our health, even fruit and vegetables – overeat carrots and they turn your skin orange. The DASH way of eating is about sensible portions of freshly made, home-cooked meals, with a focus on plant proteins. Although meat – and even processed meats – are part of this way of eating, it is within the context of balance and moderation. Meat is not bad for our health, but it is better for the environment if we choose to eat less of it and move to more sustainable plant proteins. Choosing meat that is free-range and locally farmed will help reduce your carbon footprint; it can be more expensive, but you will be eating less of it.

There are now many lower fat meat options available to buy and, in fact, over the years, meat has become leaner. When shopping, always choose the leanest option that you can. Loin, sirloin and tenderloin are all lean cuts, or look for the word 'select' and the percentage of fat on the food label.

When you are back at home, make sure you trim off any visible white fat, and grill your meat rather than frying it.

Vegetarians and vegans are often said to be healthier than meat eaters, with a lower risk of stroke, cholesterol levels and blood pressure.[9] Now, there is an element of truth in this, but it does depend on how you eat. A plant-based diet can be very nutritious and bring added health benefits; however, it can also be packed with ultra-processed food and miss out on some vital nutrients. If you do not eat any meat or fish, then you do need to plan and think about where you will get your intake of iron, vitamin B_{12}, selenium, omega-3s and zinc from.

Plant proteins incorporate beans and pulses, including lentils, nuts, seeds, tofu, soya mince, seitan (wheat gluten), tempeh and plant-based milks (soy, rice, oat and nut). Having a range of proteins and grains in your diet should ensure you get all those essential amino acids. If you are not used to cooking and eating plant proteins, it can take a bit of experimentation and time to get used to them. Beans and pulses are rich in soluble fibre, which can lead to some bloating and wind, so it is advisable to build up your tolerance. One way to do this is to have meals that are half meat and half beans or pulses. Aim to include a variety of proteins over your week and see the recipes and meal plans in chapters 6 and 7 for inspiration.

Fish also brings its own health benefits. Remember: the omega-3s in oily fish can help lower blood pressure, benefit heart health and reduce levels of inflammatory markers in the body. Most fish and seafood is low in fat, so makes a great choice when you are eating out. And let's not forget about eggs: once thought to be a cause of high cholesterol, we now know that it is perfectly safe to eat 1–2 eggs daily.

The take-home message: it is key to eat protein daily and to get this from a range of sources. If you like meat, then great, continue to eat it – but make sure it's lean, and be mindful of the portion sizes.

Salt

For millions of years, humans ate very small amounts of salt (0.1–1g per day), with meat being the saltiest food.[10] Salt became a preservative for food around 5,000 years ago. This led to it becoming of great economic importance as it helped keep food over the winter. Now it is used in cooking, seasoning and preserving food around the world. Over 75 per cent of our daily salt intake comes from processed foods, so those are the foods we need to reduce. Following the DASH diet should mean that this happens naturally.

In the UK, it is recommended that adults eat no more than 6g salt per day, but over the years our food has become saltier. It may come as no surprise that the majority of the population eats too much salt. In 2018–2019, the average daily salt intake in the UK was found to be 8.4g, 9.2g for men and 7.6g for women, which is 40 per cent higher than the daily recommendation.[11] This is pretty concerning when there is convincing scientific research dating back over 20 years that shows us that reducing salt intake will reduce blood pressure, which will reduce the risk of heart disease and stroke!

One such study gave people with raised blood pressure 12g, 6g and 3g salt per day. Those eating 3g salt had the greatest change in their blood pressure: it reduced the furthest and was still like this one year later.[12] Good news – eating less salt can reduce your blood pressure long term. In fact, a summary of the research in this area concluded that a reduction to less than 5–6g of salt per day would lower the blood pressure enough to reduce stroke deaths by about one-quarter (24 per cent) and death from heart disease by one-fifth (20 per cent).[13]

Sodium versus salt

Salt is 40 per cent sodium and 60 per cent chloride, but you only really need to worry about sodium. The terms salt and sodium can be used interchangeably on food labels. While salt does increase blood pressure, we need some of it in our diet, as it plays an important role in the body. Sodium helps nerves and muscles to function correctly and is also needed to help the body regulate water and fluid balance. Too much sodium, though, and blood pressure increases. We see in population studies that blood pressures are lower in tribes eating lower salt diets. Of course, there can be many other factors at play here, but the amount of evidence does suggest salt plays a major role.[14] The Intersalt study was a large international study that found there was a link between salt intake and blood pressure, and that lowering sodium intake by 100mmol was associated with a 3mmHg reduction in systolic blood pressure.

> **'How do I convert sodium to salt?'**
>
> Convert from milligrams (mg) of sodium to grams (g) of salt by multiplying the sodium quantity by 2.5 and then dividing by 1,000. For example, to calculate how much salt equals 2,500mg sodium, you would do the following:
>
> 2,500 x 2.5 = 6,250 ÷ 1,000 = 6.25g
>
> Therefore, 2,500mg sodium = 6.25g salt

The standard DASH diet focused on no more than 3,000mg sodium per day, which is equal to 7.5g salt (1½ teaspoons). This is more than the recommended amount in the UK these days, but due to the combination of the whole eating plan, this was shown to be highly effective. Taking this further, the researchers decided to look in finer detail at salt. Another study went on comparing the control diet and the DASH diet for 30 days at three levels of salt intake: 3,000mg sodium (1½ teaspoons salt), 2,400mg sodium (1¼ teaspoons salt) and 1,500mg sodium (¾ teaspoon salt) per day. The participants all then switched, so each person tried each level of salt intake. Reducing salt intake had extra benefits on lowering blood pressure on both the control and DASH diet. The lowest salt diet, at 1,500mg sodium (¾ teaspoon salt) per day, combined with the DASH diet had the greater benefits and reduced blood pressure even further.[15] There is no need to be counting up all the salt you eat in the day: the main message is to focus on eating less of it.

The DASH diet is usually naturally lower in salt, as you eat more fruit and vegetables, leaving less room for salty snacks. What happens when you combine the DASH diet with salt reduction too? Well, you get added benefits![16] While we know that following the DASH diet alone will lower your blood pressure, when you eat less salt and follow the DASH diet, you get the combined effects: a double whammy. The research has looked into this with interesting findings. Using six diet groups, they gave people a normal diet, a high sodium diet, or a low sodium diet for 30 days and did the same with people on the DASH diet. After 30 days, the groups were switched around to a diet with a different salt content. The results showed that although reducing salt intake led to improvements in blood pressure for the normal and DASH diets, there were greater reductions for those on the DASH diet.[17] This tells us that, while eating a lower salt diet should help you reduce your blood pressure, if you do it in conjunction with the DASH diet, you will get even better results. The good news is that while following the DASH diet, you are likely to be cooking more from scratch and will instantly be avoiding pre-packaged snack foods, so hopefully eating less salt will be second nature.

DASH-SODIUM TRIAL (N.I.H.)

All participants (N=412

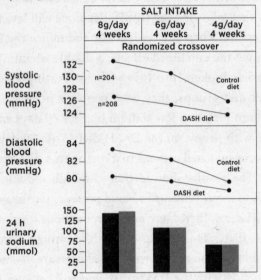

Figure 1. Changes in blood pressure and 24-hour urinary sodium excretion with the reduction in salt intake in all participants (hypertensives: n=169; normotensives: n=243) on the normal American diet (i.e. control diet) and on DASH diet. (Redrawn from Sacks 2001). Taken from actiononsalt.org.uk

Reducing your salt intake

The salt in our diet comes largely from snack foods, bread, pre-made meals and the salt we add into our meals.[18] As a general rule, if you are eating more fruit, vegetables and wholegrains, and less refined carbohydrates, then you will end up reducing your salt intake. Eating this way will also mean that you need to cook more meals from scratch, so with a few small tweaks to your cooking, your whole diet can become lower in salt.

Make sure you watch out for salty foods, such as stock cubes, soy sauce, anchovies, bacon, cheese, gravy granules, olives, pickles, salami and cured meats, salted nuts, smoked meat and fish, baked beans, canned spaghetti, yeast extract, bread, pasta sauce, crisps, pizza, ready meals, canned soup, pre-packaged sandwiches, sausages, tomato ketchup, mayonnaise and sauces, and breakfast cereals.

Where possible, choose low-salt or no-added-salt versions of foods. Check the ingredients label for salt, sodium, monosodium glutamate (MSG), garlic salt, sea salt, Himalayan salt and celery salt. These are all still salt.

Tips for cooking with less salt:

- Use low-salt stock cubes or make your own stock by boiling the bones from your chicken/meat carcass or vegetable peelings.
- Remove the salt cellar from the table! Instead, keep fresh herbs and dried chilli flakes there to add flavour to meals.
- Look for low-salt options of canned foods and sauces. Condiments including mustard, ketchup, Worcestershire sauce, soy sauce, teriyaki sauce and relish can all be salty.
- Rinse all canned beans, pulses and lentils and tuna to help remove the salt. You can soak and cook dried beans as well. This is cheaper than buying the canned versions.

- Make your own soup instead of using cans.
- Cut down on smoked and cured meats, hot dog sausages and processed meats.
- Reduce the number of takeaways, ready meals and ultra-processed foods that you eat.
- There is no need to add salt to many dishes when you are cooking; instead, add plenty of fresh herbs and spices for flavour.
- Limit olives, capers and pickled vegetables.
- Check seasoning mixes, such as fajitas and meat rubs, as these can be salty.
- Check with your doctor/dietitian before switching to a salt substitute, as these can contain higher potassium levels that can interfere with your medications.
- Check the label of ready-made foods you buy and choose the lower salt option. As a guide, less than 0.3g salt (0.1g sodium) per 100g is a little, and over 1.5g salt (0.6g sodium) per 100g is a lot.[19]

	Low	Medium	High
Salt	0–0.3g	0.3–1.5g	More than 1.5g
Sodium	0–0.1g	0.1–0.6g	More than 0.6g

Reading a food label

It is a great skill to know how to read a food label. You will mainly be cooking from scratch, but that doesn't mean you won't be buying processed foods. Let's not forget that a can of chopped tomatoes is processed! Processed foods are not necessarily bad for us: some are not recommended in large amounts in our diets, but others, like chopped tomatoes, may be items we eat almost daily. So, when you are shopping, how do you know which food item to choose? The key is to look at the labels.

	High	Low
Salt	>1.5g salt/100g (0.6g sodium)	0.3g salt/100g (0.1g sodium)
Sugar	>22.5g sugar/100g	5g sugar/100g
Saturated fat	>5g saturated fat/100g	3g saturated fat/100g

1. Often, food labels are written per 100g, which is really useful for comparing items. Check out the saturated fat, salt and sugar content per 100g. How do they compare to the figures above?
2 Look at the portion size or at how many servings are in a packet. A food may seem very high in

saturated fat/salt/sugar per 100g, but then you may only need a small amount of it.

3. I don't encourage people to get hung up on the calories contained in a food, but instead to look at the nutrients and ingredients. You can have something that is high in calories and packed full of nutrients, such as nuts, or something high in calories, such as cake. There is nothing wrong with either food, but we want to eat nuts more often and keep cake for less frequent occasions.

4. Check out what is in a food by reading the ingredients list. Look out for hydrogenated/trans fats, sugar, any type of syrup, honey, molasses, fructose and salt. The ingredients have to be listed in order of weight, from highest to lowest. As an example, if rice syrup is the second ingredient in a cereal bar, then that will be a very sweet snack.

5

Lifestyle Advice

While your daily nutrition plays a hugely important role in your health, there are other lifestyle factors that you can alter too. Alcohol, smoking, stress reduction and, of course, exercise are other key areas to think about. Once again, goal setting is the key. You may not be able to work on every area at once, so make a plan about where to start, then build on it. Realism is also paramount. Snacking, eating out and enjoying the occasional takeaway can be part of life; below are some top tips to help you navigate these areas.

Alcohol intake

The original DASH diet study kept alcohol to two drinks or fewer a day. Drinking more than the recommended 14 units of alcohol per week is well known as a risk factor that can increase the chances of high blood pressure. This doesn't mean you have to stop drinking, but it is good to reassess how much you drink in a week and look at how much a unit really is. Aim to have several alcohol-free days a week, and limit your intake to up to two units a day if you are male, and up to one unit a day if you are female. A standard unit is one small glass of wine or half a pint of beer or lager. However, it does depend on the strength of the drink. If a drink has a higher alcohol percentage or ABV (alcohol by volume), then reduce your serving size accordingly. For example, a strong pint of lager can be three units, and a weaker lager two units. Here is a great tool for working out your alcohol units: https://alcoholchange.org.uk/alcohol-facts/interactive-tools/unit-calculator

Smoking

When you smoke, it creates an environment that makes it easier for cholesterol to stick to the lining of the arteries. It is said that within 20 minutes of stopping your last cigarette, your blood pressure and pulse decrease. Smoking is known to increase the risk of lung cancer as well as heart attack or stroke. Stopping smoking is a definite win for your health.

Eating out/takeaways

Most restaurants serve large portions of main meals and can be low on the vegetable portions, making eating out trickier. Here are some key tricks and tips for making it healthier:

1. BE MENU SAVVY – Read the menu and look for those DASH diet-friendly meals. This is getting easier with the rise in plant-based eating, as there are more vegetarian and vegan options. Or look for your favourite meals and for sides you can swap in

to make them more DASH-friendly. Aim for the vegetable-laden dishes or order extra sides. At some places, you can get a wonderful selection of side dishes instead of a main meal. Why not order a meat or fish starter and pair it with some vegetable sides? Or add extra vegetable toppings to a pizza? Or swap onion rings for a portion of your favourite vegetable?

2 SHARING IS CARING – If you are eating out with someone, why not share a meat main and order a mix of vegetables/large side salad? If they don't want to share a main meal, then ask them to just share the accompaniments.

3 PORTION CAUTION – When you eat out or order in, you usually get larger portions than you need. Ask to take part of the meal home (divide the carbohydrates into half on your plate) or ask for a smaller portion, as some places will do reduced-size meals.

4 BEWARE BREAD BASKETS – These are extra carbohydrates and probably not wholegrain. Ask to have the bread basket removed once you have had some, or ask them not to bring it in the first place.

5. WATCH THE DRESSINGS – These can be high in saturated fat, sugar and salt. Ask for the dressing on the side so you can choose how much you need. Ask if there is a low-fat dressing option, or if you can just have olive oil and balsamic vinegar on a salad.

Takeaways are often high in salt, saturated fat and sugar, but that does not mean you have to totally avoid them. As I've mentioned before, no food is off limits, so this includes takeaways. It is all about how you add to the dish. Can you cook your own brown rice to go with a curry and order vegetable sides, or cook a vegetable curry at home? Have a side salad with a pizza and keep your portion smaller. Corn on the cob, peas and baked beans make quick additions to a burger meal. Many places will have a grilled chicken option: just add some salad and a wholemeal pitta/roll, and there's a DASH meal for you.

Travelling can also make it tricky to stick to DASH meals. Instead of striving for perfection, go for a little preparation and some self-kindness. If you can't eat all your portions in a day, that's ok. Take fruit and snacks with you, look for a skimmed latte for your low-fat dairy, and add salads to your meals. When you arrive somewhere new, find the local food shop and stock up on nuts, low-fat cheese, fruit and veggies.

Snack attack

Snacking can often be the time when people struggle to stick to a healthy eating plan.

If you are consistently not managing to meet the portions of a certain food group, then add it to your snacks. Remember, planning is key. Think about why you are not managing to eat it – is it that you don't like it? Are you eating something else instead? Or are you just too busy and forgetting? What can you do to make that food enjoyable and part of your routine?

Mid-afternoon snack time can be a time that people nosedive into the biscuit tin. Make sure you plan to have DASH-friendly choices available. You could make up some snack balls by food-processing nuts, seeds and dried fruit together. Roll the mixture into balls and they will freeze well or keep in an airtight container for a few days. See some simple snack recipes in the recipe section (see pages 149–157), including flapjacks, smoothies and energy balls.

Fruit alone as a snack is perfectly fine, but it can leave you hungry soon after. This might not be a problem if it is nearly a mealtime; however, if you need your snack to keep you going for longer, then add in some protein or a high-fibre food.

Here are some snack ideas, depending on your requirements:

Fruit/Veg	Protein	Fibre
Carrots/peppers	Hummus	
Apple	Nuts	
Grapes	Cheese	
Pear	Latte	
Berries	Yogurt	
Satsumas		Wholegrain crackers
Banana	Nut butters	
Dried apricots	Unsalted nuts	
Apple		Popcorn

Other heart-healthy behaviours

Many of the risk factors for heart diseases can be reduced by making dietary and lifestyle changes as outlined in this book. Focusing on a diet that puts an emphasis on a balanced way of eating, eating more plant foods, stopping smoking and being active are all things that can help.

Weight loss

If you have been diagnosed with high blood pressure, then you may well have been told that you should try and lose weight. This is because there is a correlation between central obesity (carrying weight around your tummy) and high blood pressure. Much of the research on high blood pressure has shown a relationship with body weight.[1] If you are obese, losing weight may help your blood pressure decrease and so lower your risk of heart diseases. However, the key is to lose weight and keep it off rather than yoyo dieting.[2]

So, should you be trying to lose weight while you're on the DASH diet? Weight loss may be beneficial for some people, but it isn't helpful to make it your main focus. Instead, look at your overall lifestyle patterns, and try to add in healthy behaviours. For example, if you eat more fruit and vegetables, you will have less space in your diet for cakes and biscuits. It doesn't mean that you cannot eat those foods, but it is all about that balance.

As always, it is important to look at the science. Studies on the DASH diet show that the benefits of lowered blood pressure are seen whether you lose weight or not. So, if you do not feel you need to lose weight, then you can still get the benefits. Weight loss does not have to be part of this way of eating. For some people, weight loss may either be a side effect or something that is a helpful part of lifestyle change; however, let's not forget that slim people can also develop high blood pressure, so it is certainly not essential for all those with high blood pressure to lose weight.

If you have been told you should lose weight, though, then the DASH diet should help you with that, without it becoming a main focus. Losing weight and successfully keeping it off comes from making lasting lifestyle changes, which is what the DASH diet is all about.

It is common in the medical profession to use a person's body mass index (BMI) as a way to gauge their health and weight; however, this is only a very rough guide. Devised by a mathematician in the 1830s, the body mass index is a measure of your weight in kilograms divided by your squared height in metres. So, if you weigh 65kg (143lb) and are 165cm (5 feet, 4 inches) tall, you can work out your BMI using the following calculation:

$65 \div (1.65 \times 1.65) = 23.9$
Therefore, your BMI is 23.9

In general terms, a BMI of 19–25 is a healthy weight, 26–30 is overweight and 31–39 is obese. However, many people can have a higher BMI and be perfectly healthy, while others can have a lower BMI and suffer health conditions. So using BMI as the only way to judge your health is not an accurate measure. It is important to use some common sense when looking at BMI, and consider it in combination with other measures, such as waist circumference (below), a full physical from your GP and a detailed dietary assessment.

One way to check if you have central obesity is to measure your waist circumference. Carrying more fat around your middle can be a risk factor for chronic diseases, including heart disease, so if your waist is 94cm (37 inches) or more for men, or 80cm (31½ inches) or more for women, the DASH diet may enable you to lose some of that tummy fat.

If you are overweight and feel it would be helpful, then there is evidence to show that weight loss of 1kg (2lb 4oz) can lead to 1mmHg reduction in systolic blood pressure (the top number).[3] The problem with focusing solely on weight loss, though, is it becomes a short-term goal and the quality of your diet can suffer. Nutrition is so important, and we know many of the foods in the DASH diet are essential for heart health, so cutting calories is not the answer. Instead of making weight loss your focus, I recommend you stick to the DASH diet guidelines in this book. If it is needed, you may find that some secondary weight loss occurs naturally as you alter your eating and activity levels.

The research shows that if you are overweight/obese, adding exercise and weight loss to the DASH diet can lead to even larger reductions in blood pressure, but don't forget that you can still get benefits without the weight loss.[4] If you do feel that you need to lose weight, then slow and steady is the best way. Losing weight too fast can feel good intially, but you will be losing fluid first, and then muscle rather than fat. The optimal rate of weight loss for losing fat is 500g–1kg (1lb 2oz–2lb 4oz) per week. I wouldn't recommend that you start with a lower calorie DASH diet plan. Instead, transition slowly. Start by focusing on the plan that your body needs, so 2,000kcals for a woman and 2,500kcals for a man. See how this feels: how hungry are you? How full are you? Are you managing to eat all your portions? Alongside this, add in some activity that you enjoy and let your mind and body adapt to this new lifestyle. After a few weeks, if you are not seeing a change in your weight, think about whether there are other changes in terms of your overall health. Try not to overly restrict your eating: this is not a fad diet, but a lifestyle change. It will take time to see the long-term benefits. Why not just jump straight in to a lower calorie eating plan? Well, we want this to be long term, not another crash diet. You need to feel satisfied, full and nourished, rather than being left wanting more. Making changes to your way of eating also requires some determination, planning and time, so going step by step will be kinder to your body and mind.

Another crude way to work out which DASH plan to follow is to roughly calculate your energy needs (see table, page 86). Now, this is very rough, but it does provide a general guide to the calories you need to maintain your weight. To lose weight, you need to reduce your eating by 500kcals, or eat less and exercise more. It is not recommended that you reduce your usual calorie intake by more than 500kcals. Eating too few calories will make it impossible to get all those DASH portions into your day, and so you will not get the heart-healthy benefits. It can also affect your energy levels, physical wellbeing and mental health.

Roughly calculating your energy needs

Activity Level	Kcals per 1kg (2lb 4oz) body weight
Sedentary	30
Moderate	35
Heavy	40

Exercise

Being active can also help with blood pressure reduction and improve your cardiovascular health by exercising your heart and blood vessels. Exercise is also a wonderful mood booster, helping you to deal with stress and increasing your energy levels. Nowadays, many people have sedentary jobs where they sit all day, then travel home and sit more there. Compare this to 50–80 years ago, when there were many more active jobs, fewer cars and less equipment to help us do everyday tasks. You would have been squatting down, bending, reaching and carrying more. Back then, you wouldn't have needed to do planned exercise, as it was all part of a normal day.

In this current age, we do need to plan activity into our day, whether that is walking to work, going to the gym or running about in the park with the kids – it all counts. Aim to be active for 150 minutes or more a week. The key is to find activities that you really enjoy, and also to find ways to just be more active in your daily life. Build in a walking meeting, stand up and move about when on the phone, and factor in some stretches while you wait for the kettle to boil! You also want to exercise at a moderate intensity for some sessions of 10 minutes or longer at a time. This can simply be done via fast walking or walking up and down stairs. Check that your heart rate is elevated and your body is getting warmer, but that you can still talk.[5] Exercise really doesn't need any fancy equipment; your own body can be the weights.

Improving your fitness levels can help reduce your blood pressure, your cholesterol levels and your risk of developing type 2 diabetes. Some health and life insurance policies now monitor your activity as a way to reduce your premium. A simple way to measure how active you are is to use an activity tracker. This will give you feedback on how many steps you do and how many minutes you are active for. Although 10,000 steps is often used as a guide, this concept was actually a marketing strategy to sell pedometers; there is little science to support that particular step count and there is no one-size-fits-all figure. Monitor your activity throughout a week. See how many minutes of exercise you do, and perhaps how many steps you take. It is all relative, so any increase in your activity and step count will be beneficial. A 2010 study showed a 10 per cent decrease in the risk of metabolic syndrome (this is a combination of symptoms that increases your risk of diabetes and heart disease – see page 29) per 1,000 extra steps per day.[6] The bottom line is to build an active lifestyle so it becomes part of what you do and is an enjoyable part of your life.

Some ways to build activity into your daily life:

- Walk as much as you can, whether that is to work, to the shops, or on the school run. It soon adds up in terms of your steps, and it is great to be outside, plus it helps the environment. If you can't walk the full distance, then drive part of the way and park.
- Take the stairs instead of a lift whenever you can. It has become a well-known part of our family life that Mum always chooses the stairs!
- Try to find time to be active BEFORE you relax or sit down at home, otherwise you will get too comfy and want to switch off. Maybe build in some activity on the way home from work or first thing in the morning.
- Make time for some movement at lunchtime, such as a walk around the block. This can also help to wake you up ready for the afternoon.
- Keep those cans of baked beans handy (for gentle weightlifting, not eating!) and do some resistance work while cooking dinner!

There is some evidence that suggests combining the DASH diet with resistance training brings extra benefits in terms of losing fat.[7] Resistance training can seem intimidating to start with, but a simple routine with squats, using cans of baked beans for weights, is something simple you can do at home. A 10-week study on a small group of overweight and obese people in their sixties tried adding resistance training to advice on the DASH diet. The group doing the resistance training reduced their BMI, percentage of body fat and fat mass, plus some reductions were seen in blood tests for coronary heart disease markers.[8] Check with your doctor that you are cleared for exercise first, and do seek out a trained professional to advise you on where to start.

Motivation can be a sticking point with exercise. If you haven't done any exercise for a while, or know you are not very motivated right now, then you could seek out a personal trainer to advise you, or ask a friend to start walking with you. For many people, exercising with friends or in a group class can make it far easier to stick to and more enjoyable. This can very much be a personality thing. If you are a social creature, then you will probably want to be with others –or you may enjoy team sports. Also, think through where you like to exercise: outdoors in nature, in a small studio, being part of a larger gym, etc. Think back to things that you used to enjoy doing, or consider whether there is something you have always wanted to try. Buying some workout clothes that you love or a good pair of comfy walking shoes can also make you feel more comfortable and help with the exercise that you choose to do. Check out the timetable in your local gym, look on social media for a netball group, martial arts lessons or a dance class, or look locally for a small studio offering Pilates and yoga. Whatever you choose, make it something you can commit to doing regularly and enjoy.

Motivation

We know that when people take part in a research study, it doesn't always mimic normal life. In the original DASH research, everyone was provided with all their meals and told exactly what to eat and drink. They had motivational sessions and dietitians to keep them on track. It is definitely easier to stick to a healthy lifestyle when you have it all planned for you and someone cheering you on. In real life, though, you have to be your own cheerleader!

The Premier study looked at what would happen if you were given one of three levels of support to complement the eating plan:

Group 1) one education session
Group 2) 18 education sessions over six months
Group 3) 18 sessions plus advice on the DASH diet

All three groups had improvements in blood pressure, but not to the same extent as those participants who had been given the food pre-prepared. The group given advice on the DASH diet had the best improvements: in fact, 77 per cent of people in this group who started with hypertension ended the study with normal blood pressure.[9] Even those who were just given one education session still saw significant improvements in their blood pressure, which could have been due to knowing they were in a study and were being monitored. So, what does this tell us? Having your meals pre-prepared for you makes it easier to stick to a new way of eating, which is obvious, but not practical for many of us. Not many people can afford a personal chef, but there are meal delivery services you can sign up to. They are more expensive than cooking from scratch, but could certainly help you in the short term while you get started. Personally, I think some of the benefit of making this long-term lifestyle change is learning how to plan meals, prepare food and cook from scratch.

Having someone to hold you accountable can make a huge difference to staying on board with lifestyle changes. This is unlikely to be your doctor, as appointment slots are usually short, so consider finding a dietitian to work with at the beginning. Having a monthly check-in session can be hugely beneficial for tips, motivation and advice, and to help you remember to stick to the plan. There are dietitians working around the UK in the NHS and private practice. Always check credentials, as there is a difference between a nutritionist, a dietitian and a nutritional therapist. Dietitians are the only ones trained in managing medical conditions with nutrition. Alternatively, look for a life coach or therapist to help you with the motivation side of things, or find a friend or family member who can support you or even make the changes with you.

Lowering your stress levels

Modern life is stressful. The stress that we feel in our bodies has an impact on our general health. We have two nervous systems, the autonomic and the peripheral. The autonomic nervous system can function in two ways: as the sympathetic or parasympathetic nervous system. As a general rule, the sympathetic nervous system is your 'fight or flight' system that is there to protect us when our bodies have a problem. The parasympathetic nervous system helps us to 'rest and digest'.

If we are living in a state of constant stress, the body may not digest food properly or relax. While we are designed to be able to run away from danger, we are not designed to live under constant stress. Another key factor in managing your blood pressure is finding ways to lower your stress levels. It may not be possible to live a completely stress-free life, and this is perfectly fine: the body is designed to live with a certain level of stress. However, when we are living under constant stress, or too much of it, the body will suffer. Think about how much stress you are currently feeling on a daily basis. How could you reduce it or help to manage it? Simple strategies such as breathing, meditation and regular walking, yoga or Pilates can all help.

Where to go from here

As a result of our walk through the DASH diet, I hope you have been inspired to make some lasting changes to your lifestyle. Adding in more fruit, vegetables and wholegrains may feel like hard work to start with, but the health benefits are so very worthwhile.

Remember to start small: plan a few key changes that you can begin with and work on those, then build on your success. This is not a short-term fix, but a long-term lifestyle change; it is OK to take your time over it, just as long as you keep focused and continue to make further changes. Setting out a list of your goals with a timescale in which you aim to achieve them is an ideal way to do this.

This is not a diet – I repeat, not a diet! It may go off-course at times, but that is a part of life – there is no failure, just more chances to make changes and learn. Things might not to go according to plan all the time. When this happens, you just need to adjust your plan and move forward. Seek out those who can encourage you to keep going and use the recipes and meal plans in the book as your starting point (see chapters 6 and 7). Completing those three-week meal plans a couple of times over should help you adapt to your new way of life. I do hope you get lasting health benefits and lifelong wellness from the DASH diet.

6

The Recipes

In this section, you will find a selection of recipes that I hope you will find helpful as you start on the DASH diet. The recipes have been divided into Breakfasts, Lunches, Dinners, and Snacks, Sides & Sweet Nibbles, but you can mix and match. For instance, some of the lunches could be served with a side dish to make a great dinner; some breakfasts could also be used for lunch, and vice versa! There are no strict rules here – these are all meant to be ideas to get you started. A top tip is to make an extra serving of dinner so you can have the leftovers for lunch the next day.

I've noted down the rough portions of fruit and vegetables per serving for each recipe. These do not include any of the serving suggestions, so where a meal includes the suggestion of a side salad, you can count that as an extra portion of vegetables. As an example, the Homemade Falafel Wraps (see page 123) provide you with two portions of vegetables, but add the salad leaves they're served with, and that's three portions.

The recipes have been planned for the 2,000kcal meal plan. You will see asterisks in brackets (*) alongside some of the ingredient measurements. These are larger portion sizes for those following the 2,500kcal meal plan. If you are following the 1,600kcal plan, then please adjust the portions accordingly (for example, using smaller portions of wholegrains). Remember, these are just a guide and I am not advocating that you count calories on a daily basis. Instead, focus on tuning into your hunger and fullness cues, and use the portion guidance as a way to educate yourself on what a normal amount should be. We all have days when we eat more and days when we eat less; that is normal.

Breakfasts

Tropical Fruit Cup

1 serving (2 portions of fruit per serving)

3 tablespoons frozen mango flesh, defrosted and
    chopped
2 canned pineapple slices in fruit juice, drained
    and chopped
150ml (¼ pint) natural yogurt
3 tablespoons low-sugar granola (*5 tablespoons)
1 teaspoon pumpkin seeds

In a tall serving glass, arrange the fruit, yogurt and granola in
layers. Sprinkle the pumpkin seeds on top.

This can be eaten immediately or chilled in the refrigerator
for a couple of hours before serving.

Overnight Oats with Mixed Berries

1 serving (2 portions of fruit per serving)

50g (1¾oz) rolled oats (*65g/2½oz)
1 tablespoon chia seeds
1 tablespoon raisins
3 tablespoons fresh mixed berries (such as
    raspberries, blueberries and strawberries)
150ml (¼ pint) semi-skimmed or skimmed milk

Layer up the oats, chia seeds and raisins in a cereal bowl or a
suitable airtight container/tub (if you are taking it to work).
Top with the berries and pour over the milk.

Cover and leave to soak in the refrigerator overnight.

Grab the oats the next morning to eat at home or at work.

Greek Yogurt with Fruit & Nuts

1 serving (1 portion of fruit per serving)

150ml (¼ pint) Greek yogurt

30g (1oz) unsalted mixed nuts of your choice
(such as almonds and walnuts)

3 tablespoons fresh mixed fruit (such as banana,
strawberries and mango)

Mix the yogurt, nuts and berries together in a bowl and serve.

Make Your Own Muesli

10 servings (1 portion of fruit per serving)

500g (1lb 2oz) rolled oats

250g (9oz) mixed dried fruit (such as raisins,
chopped dried apricots, chopped dried apple
rings, banana chips and coconut flakes)

5 tablespoons mixed seeds (such as pumpkin
and sunflower)

100g (3½oz) mixed unsalted nuts (such as
almonds, pecans and walnuts)

fresh fruit and semi-skimmed or skimmed milk,
to serve

Mix the oats, dried fruit, seeds and nuts together in a large bowl,
then transfer to an airtight container. This muesli will keep for
several weeks in a cool, dry place.

Use a measuring cup to scoop out your portions, serving
¾–1 cup (40–65g/1½–2½oz) per portion.

Serve with a portion of fresh fruit and some milk.

Many ready-made mueslis are high in sugar, expensive and contain ingredients you may not like, so why not make your own? It's quick, easy, delicious – and more economical too!

Porridge with Apple & Cinnamon

1 serving (1 portion of fruit per serving)

50g (1¾oz) rolled oats (*65g/2½oz)
1 tablespoon flaxseeds (linseeds)
1 tablespoon raisins
150ml (¼ pint) semi-skimmed or skimmed milk
1 dessert apple, cored and grated (no need
   to peel)
1 teaspoon ground cinnamon
1 tablespoon Greek yogurt

Place the oats, flaxseeds (linseeds), raisins and milk in a heatproof bowl. Stir, then microwave on high, uncovered, for around 1 minute (this will depend on the power of your microwave) or until the porridge reaches the desired consistency. Stir in the grated apple, sprinkle the cinnamon on top, then microwave for a further 30 seconds, if desired, depending on how you like your porridge.

Alternatively, place the oats, flaxseeds (linseeds), raisins and milk in a saucepan. Simmer over a low heat for a few minutes, stirring as the mixture cooks, until the porridge reaches the desired consistency. Stir in the grated apple and sprinkle the cinnamon on top at the end of the cooking time.

Top with the Greek yogurt and serve.

Banana & Pumpkin Seed Pancakes

1 serving/3 pancakes (2 portions of fruit per serving)

1 banana, peeled
3 tablespoons rolled oats
2 teaspoons pumpkin seeds
½ teaspoon ground cinnamon
1 egg
rapeseed oil, for greasing

To serve

1 tablespoon Greek yogurt
3 tablespoons frozen mixed berries, defrosted
drizzle of maple syrup

Mash the banana in a bowl, then mix in the oats, pumpkin seeds and cinnamon.

Make space in the bowl, then crack in the egg and beat it. Mix everything together.

Lightly grease a nonstick frying pan or griddle pan with a little rapeseed oil, then heat over a medium–high heat until hot.

Drop 3 serving spoonfuls of the mixture into the hot pan and let the pancakes cook for a few minutes until they start to firm up a little and you see bubbles on the surface. When you flip the pancakes over, they should be lightly browned. (Don't turn them too soon, as they are quite delicate and may fall apart). Cook for a few minutes on the second side until lightly browned.

Transfer the cooked pancakes to a plate and serve immediately with the Greek yogurt dolloped on top, the berries scattered over, finished with a drizzle of maple syrup.

Carrot Cake Muffins

6–12 servings/Makes 12 muffins (1–2 portions of fruit/veg per serving)

250g (9oz) plain wholemeal flour

100g (3½oz) soft light brown sugar

1 tablespoon baking powder

2 teaspoons bicarbonate of soda

2 teaspoons ground cinnamon

½ teaspoon ground ginger

50g (1¾oz) raisins

175g (6oz) unsweetened apple sauce, cooled (see Tip)

3 carrots, peeled and finely grated

1 banana, peeled and mashed

50ml (2fl oz) rapeseed oil

150ml (¼ pint) natural or Greek yogurt, to serve (per serving)

Preheat the oven to 200°C (400°F), Gas Mark 6. Line a 12-cup muffin tin with muffin cases.

Sift the flour into a bowl, tipping the bran left in the sieve into the bowl too. Add the sugar, baking powder, bicarbonate of soda, cinnamon and ginger and mix together. Stir in the raisins.

In a separate bowl, combine the apple sauce, grated carrots, mashed banana and rapeseed oil. Add the wet ingredients to the dry and fold together to combine (don't overmix, or you'll end up with heavy muffins).

Carefully spoon the mixture into the muffin cases, dividing it evenly between them. Bake for 15–20 minutes or until risen and lightly browned.

Remove from the oven, transfer to a wire rack and leave to cool a little. These are best served warm, but can also be made ahead of time to grab on the go. Any leftovers will keep in an airtight container for up to 3 days. Serve 1–2 muffins with a yogurt.

To make the apple sauce, peel, core and chop a medium cooking apple. Place in a small saucepan with 120ml (4fl oz) water, cover and cook over a medium heat for 10–15 minutes or until the apple is soft and pulpy. Remove from the heat and leave to cool. If the sauce isn't smooth, blend it briefly to make a purée.

Simple Tofu Veggies on Toast

2 servings (2 portions of veg per serving)

1 tablespoon olive oil
½ onion, sliced
8 closed-cup mushrooms, trimmed and sliced
1 garlic clove, crushed
200g (7oz) baby spinach
150g (5½oz) firm tofu, drained
2 slices of wholemeal sourdough or rye bread
reduced-fat olive oil spread, for spreading

Heat the olive oil in a small frying pan over a medium–high heat. Add the onion and sauté for 5 minutes or until softened and browned. Add the mushrooms and garlic and sauté for a further 5 minutes or until softened and browned.

Stir in the spinach and cook for a minute or so until wilted, then crumble in the tofu.

Meanwhile, toast the bread on both sides, then spread with a little olive oil spread.

Serve the tofu-veggie mixture on the hot toast.

Mediterranean Veg Omelette

1 serving (2 portions of veg per serving)

1 teaspoon olive oil
large handful of baby spinach
8 cherry tomatoes, halved
1 small garlic clove, crushed
2 large eggs
1 tablespoon Greek yogurt
25g (⅘oz) feta cheese, crumbled
2 slices of wholemeal sourdough or rye bread,
  or a wholemeal pitta bread, toasted
  (*3 slices)

Heat the olive oil in a small nonstick frying pan over a medium heat. Add the spinach, cherry tomatoes and garlic and sauté for 1 minute until the spinach has wilted. Transfer the spinach mixture from the pan to a warm plate using a slotted spoon and set aside.

Beat the eggs in a small bowl, then combine them with the Greek yogurt.

Add the egg mixture to the frying pan and stir gently over a medium heat for 1 minute, then leave to set, without stirring, for a further 1–2 minutes.

Now top the omelette with the spinach mixture and sprinkle over the crumbled feta. Fold the omelette in half, slide it on to the same plate you used for the spinach mixture and serve with the bread or toasted pitta.

Eggs on Toast with Tomatoes

1 serving (2 portions of veg per serving)

2 tomatoes, chopped
½ red or yellow pepper, cored, deseeded
  and chopped
2 eggs
1 slice of wholemeal bread (*2 slices)
reduced-fat olive oil spread, for spreading
freshly ground black pepper
chopped chives, to garnish

Heat a large, nonstick frying pan over a medium heat until hot. Add the tomatoes and pepper and cook for 5 minutes, stirring occasionally, until softened.

Move the tomatoes and pepper to one side of the pan to make space for the eggs. Crack the eggs into the pan and cook for about 3 minutes, or until cooked to your liking.

Meanwhile, toast the bread on both sides, then spread with a little olive oil spread.

Serve the eggs and tomato-pepper mix on the toast. Season with black pepper and sprinkle with the chives to garnish.

Smoked Salmon Bagel

1 serving (1 portion of fruit/veg per serving)

½ wholemeal bagel (*1 bagel)
2 tablespoons cottage cheese with chives
100g (3½oz) smoked salmon
large handful of baby spinach, rocket leaves
  or watercress
glass of semi-skimmed or skimmed milk, to serve

Slice the bagel in half and toast on both sides.

Spread the toasted bagel with the cottage cheese. Top with the smoked salmon and spinach, rocket or watercress.

Serve with a glass of milk.

BLTM

1 serving (1 portion of fruit/veg per serving)

2 rindless unsmoked back bacon rashers
  or medallions
1 teaspoon olive oil
4 closed-cup mushrooms, trimmed and sliced
2 slices of wholemeal bread
1 teaspoon mustard of your choice
small handful of torn lettuce leaves or
  baby spinach
1 tomato, sliced

Start cooking the bacon in a nonstick frying pan over a medium heat. Once it is cooked on one side, which will take about 3 minutes, turn it over, then add the olive oil and sliced mushrooms to the pan as well and cook for a further 5 minutes, or until the bacon and mushrooms are cooked stirring the mushrooms occasionally.

Place the bread on a serving plate and spread with the mustard. Layer the lettuce leaves or baby spinach and tomato slices on the first slice of bread, then add the bacon and mushrooms and top with the second slice of bread. Serve immediately.

Lunches

Green Veg Minestrone Soup

4 servings (2 portions of veg per serving)

100g (3½oz) dried wholewheat pasta (small
   pasta, such as macaroni, conchiglie, or small
   fusilli, works best) (*300g/10½oz)
1 low-salt stock cube
700ml (1¼ pints) boiling water
240g (8½oz) prepped mixed green vegetables
   (broad beans, peas, broccoli florets, soybeans/
   edamame beans, asparagus spears and green
   beans all work well)
6 spring onions, thinly sliced
400g (14oz) can cannellini or butter beans
   in water, drained and rinsed
200g (7oz) baby spinach
1 tablespoon green pesto
freshly ground black pepper

Cook the pasta in a pan of boiling water according to the packet instructions until al dente, then drain and set aside.

When the pasta is nearly cooked, crumble the stock cube into a measuring jug, pour over the measured boiling water and stir.

Place the prepped green veggies and spring onions in a separate saucepan over a medium heat and pour over the stock. Bring to the boil, then reduce the heat to a simmer. Cook for 5 minutes or until the veg are cooked and tender. (You can use frozen mixed green vegetables, if you prefer – just reduce the cooking time a little.)

Stir in the cooked pasta, beans and baby spinach, and simmer gently just to warm the beans through and wilt the spinach. Remove from the heat, stir in the pesto, season with black pepper and serve.

To make this recipe suitable for vegetarians, just use vegetable stock and a vegetarian pesto (one that doesn't include Parmesan).

White Bean and Pepper Nachos

2 servings (3 portions of veg per serving)

flesh from 1 ripe avocado
½ x 400g (14oz) can white beans in water (such as cannellini)
2 tablespoons lemon juice
1 tomato, finely diced
½ red onion, finely diced
1 red pepper, roasted (from a jar or homemade, see Tip), cored, deseeded (if homemade) and finely chopped
2 tablespoons canned (or frozen, defrosted) salt-free sweetcorn kernels
2 teaspoons olive oil
2 teaspoons red wine vinegar
2 wholemeal tortilla wraps (*4 wraps)
freshly ground black pepper
green salad, to serve

Mash the avocado flesh and white beans together in a bowl with the lemon juice to make a dip, then season to taste with black pepper. Set aside.

To make the salsa, combine the tomato, red onion, red pepper and sweetcorn in a separate bowl, then dress with the olive oil and red wine vinegar. Set aside.

Cut the wraps into triangles and then toast in a nonstick frying pan over a medium heat for a couple of minutes on each side, turning once, until gently browned and crispy.

Divide the toasted tortilla chips between two serving plates. Top with the dip and salsa. Serve with a green salad.

To roast your own peppers, preheat the oven to 220°C (425°F), Gas Mark 7. Line a baking tray with greaseproof paper. Halve the peppers, cutting through their stalks. Remove the cores and seeds, but keep the stalks on. Place the peppers on the baking tray, cut side down. Roast for 30 minutes until the skins are shrivelled with blister marks or black patches. Set aside to cool, then peel off the skins (you may wish to wear gloves to do this part).

Hummus & Veggie Sandwich

1 serving (2 portions of veg per serving)

2 slices of wholemeal bread (*3 slices)
2 tablespoons hummus (see Tip)
   (*2½ tablespoons)
large handful of mixed salad leaves
1 tomato, sliced
½ carrot, peeled and grated

Place the bread slices on a plate and spread with the hummus.

Top with the salad leaves, tomato slices and grated carrot, then either serve as an open sandwich, or sandwich the bread slices together to make a standard sandwich.

Use either shop-bought hummus or make your own (see recipe on page 151).

Egg Mayo Sandwich

1 serving (2 portions of veg per serving)

1 egg, at room temperature (*2 eggs)
1 tablespoon low-fat mayonnaise (*2 tablespoons)
½ tablespoon Greek yogurt (*1 tablespoon)
3 tablespoons canned (or frozen, defrosted)
   sweetcorn kernels
pinch of paprika
reduced-fat olive oil spread, for spreading
2 slices of wholemeal bread (*3 slices)
large handful of salad leaves
8 cherry tomatoes, halved
freshly ground black pepper

Add the egg(s) to a small pan of cold water and bring to the boil, then boil gently for 7–10 minutes for hard-boiled egg(s). Drain, then plunge the egg(s) into cold water to stop them cooking, and leave to cool. Once cool, drain and peel off the shells.

Cut up or mash the egg(s) in a small bowl, then mix with the mayo, yogurt, sweetcorn, paprika and some black pepper to taste.

Thinly spread a little reduced-fat spread over the bread slices. Top one slice of bread with the egg mayo mixture and then top with the salad leaves. Place the second slice of bread on top to make a sandwich. Place on a plate, cut in half and serve the sandwich with the cherry tomatoes on the side.

Beany Pitta Pockets

1 serving (2 portions of veg per serving)

400g (14oz) can butter beans in water, drained
and rinsed

1 tablespoon olive oil

2 tablespoons lemon juice

125g (4½oz) soft cheese

1 wholemeal pitta bread (*2 pitta breads), split
open and toasted

large handful of mixed salad leaves

1 tomato, sliced

½ cucumber, cut into sticks/batons

freshly ground black pepper

Place the beans in a food processor (or mash them well in a bowl).
Pour in the olive oil and lemon juice. Add some black pepper to
taste and whizz up (or mash together) to a smooth paste. Add the
soft cheese and whizz to combine (or mash to mix). This dip will
keep in an airtight container in the refrigerator for up to 3 days.

Fill the pitta bread with the salad leaves and add 1 tablespoon
of the butter bean dip. Serve with another tablespoon of dip on
the side, along with the tomato and cucumber.

Easy Tortilla Pizza

1 serving (2-3 portions of veg per serving)

1 wholemeal tortilla wrap (*2 wraps)
1 teaspoon tomato purée (*2 teaspoons)
½ tomato, sliced (*1 tomato)
2 closed-cup mushrooms, trimmed and sliced (*4 mushrooms)
¼ pepper (any colour), cored, deseeded and sliced (*½ pepper)
2 teaspoons canned (or frozen, defrosted) salt-free sweetcorn kernels (*4 teaspoons)
25g (⅘oz) Cheddar cheese (reduced fat, if you choose), grated (*50g/1¾oz)
mixed salad leaves, to serve

Preheat the oven to 180°C (350°F), Gas Mark 4 or preheat the grill to medium.

Spread the wrap(s) with the tomato purée and place on a baking tray. Top with the vegetables, then sprinkle the cheese over the top.

Bake for 10 minutes, or cook under the grill for a few minutes, until the cheese melts and the wrap is crispy at the edges. Serve hot, with mixed salad leaves on the side.

One Pan All-day Veggie Brunch

2 servings (2 portions of veg per serving)

½ tablespoon olive oil
1 courgette, trimmed and diced
2 tomatoes, diced

handful of mushrooms, trimmed and sliced

2 eggs (*4 eggs)

4 slices of wholegrain bread (wholegrain
    sourdough, rye or standard wholemeal)

reduced-fat olive oil spread, for spreading

Heat the olive oil in a large, nonstick frying pan with a lid. Add the courgette and cook over a medium heat for 5 minutes or until lightly browned. Now add the tomatoes and mushrooms and cook for a further 5 minutes, stirring occasionally, until all the vegetables have softened.

Make some wells in the veggies (depending on how many eggs you are using) and break in the eggs. Cover with a lid and cook for 2–3 minutes or until the whites of the eggs are cooked to your liking.

Meanwhile, spread the bread with a little reduced-fat spread.

Now serve up the all-day veggie-egg brunch with the bread, and enjoy.

Lentil Salad

2 servings (3 portions of veg per serving)

wholegrain of your choice, such as couscous,
    bulgur wheat, brown rice or freekeh (50g/1¾oz,
    75g/2¾oz or 100g/3½oz per person on
    1,600/2,000/2,500kcal meal plan)

400g (14oz) can green or brown lentils in water,
    drained and rinsed

1 red onion, finely diced

4 tomatoes, diced

½ cucumber, diced

2 large roasted red peppers (from a jar
   homemade – see Tip on page 112),
   drained and chopped

2 tablespoons olive oil

3 tablespoons cider vinegar

200g (7oz) baby spinach or mixed salad leaves

80g (2¾oz) feta cheese

small handful of mint leaves, chopped

Cook the wholegrain of your choice according to the packet instructions, then drain (if needed). Allow to cool.

Meanwhile, tip the lentils into a bowl, add the vegetables and stir. Pour over the olive oil and vinegar and toss well to mix.

Add the spinach or salad leaves, feta and mint, and mix together gently, then serve with your chosen cooked wholegrain.

The lentil salad will keep in an airtight container in the refrigerator for up to 3 days.

Mackerel & Beetroot Salad

2 servings (2 portions of veg per serving)

100g (3½oz) bulgur wheat (*150g/5½oz)

120g (4¼oz) frozen peas

1 cooked beetroot (not in vinegar), diced

2 spring onions, thinly sliced

2 tablespoons Greek yogurt

1 heaped teaspoon Dijon mustard

2 smoked mackerel fillets (each about
    125g/4½oz), skin removed
large handful of mixed salad leaves

Cook the bulgur wheat according to the packet instructions, then drain (if needed) and replace the lid to keep warm.

Meanwhile, cook the peas in a small pan of boiling water over a medium heat for 3–4 minutes (or in the microwave, according to the packet instructions) until tender, then drain.

Place the cooked peas in a bowl with the beetroot and spring onions and mix them well.

Combine the yogurt and mustard in a separate small bowl. Flake the mackerel into bite-sized pieces.

Layer the salad leaves with the beetroot and pea mix on serving plates, then top with the flaked mackerel and drizzle the yogurt sauce over. Serve.

Quick Tuna Pasta Salad

2 servings (2 portions of veg per serving)

100g (3½oz) dried wholewheat pasta, such as
    penne or fusilli (*150g/5½oz)
1 tablespoon olive oil
145g (5¼oz) can tuna in spring water
½ red onion, chopped
2 red or yellow peppers, cored, deseeded and diced
198g (7oz) can salt-free sweetcorn kernels, drained
2 tablespoons chopped parsley
1 tablespoon red wine vinegar

Cook the pasta in a pan of boiling water according to the packet instructions until al dente, then drain. Drizzle over the olive oil and toss to mix, then tip into a heatproof bowl and leave to cool.

Drain the tuna and break it into flakes using a fork. Add this to the cooled pasta along with the red onion, peppers, sweetcorn and parsley, and stir to combine. Drizzle over the red wine vinegar and toss to mix.

Serve immediately or portion into an airtight container (see Tip) and store in the refrigerator for up to 2 days.

Why not make enough for tomorrow's lunch too? This is a great recipe to make double and use in a lunchbox the next day.

Chicken & Bean Salad

2 servings (2 portions of veg per serving)

100g (3½oz) couscous (*150g/5½oz)
½ low-salt vegetable stock cube
100ml (3½fl oz) boiling water
½ red onion, thinly sliced
80g (2¾oz) cherry tomatoes, halved
1 red pepper, cored, deseeded and diced
3 heaped tablespoons (80g/2¾oz) canned (or frozen, defrosted) salt-free sweetcorn kernels
½ x 400g (14oz) can mixed beans in water, drained and rinsed
1 tablespoon olive oil
1 tablespoon balsamic vinegar
squeeze of lemon juice

200g (7oz) mixed salad leaves, shredded
100g (3½oz) cold cooked (skinless) chicken,
    chopped

Place the couscous in a medium, heatproof bowl. Crumble in the stock cube, then pour over the measured boiling water and stir. Cover with a lid or plate and leave to soak for 5–10 minutes (the couscous will absorb the liquid). Fluff it up once it's ready.

Meanwhile, mix together the red onion, tomatoes, red pepper, sweetcorn and beans in a serving bowl. Drizzle over the olive oil, vinegar and lemon juice and mix thoroughly. Add in the salad leaves, chicken and cooled couscous, and toss together to mix.

Serve immediately, or transfer to an airtight container. It will keep in the refrigerator for up to 1 day.

Dinners

Roasted Veggie Pasta

4 servings (3–4 portions of veg per serving)

1 aubergine (about 300g/10½oz), cut into
    medium chunks

1 red pepper, cored, deseeded and cut into
    medium chunks

1 yellow pepper, cored, deseeded and cut
    into medium chunks

1 red onion, cut into medium chunks

6 tomatoes, halved horizontally

2 garlic cloves, left whole with skin on

3 rosemary sprigs

2 tablespoons olive oil

dried wholewheat pasta of your choice
    (50g/1¾oz, 70g/2½oz or 100g/3½oz per person
    on 1,600/2,000/2,500kcal meal plan)

150g (5½oz) mozzarella (reduced fat, if you
    choose), drained

200g (7oz) spinach or other green leaves (such
    as kale, chard or spring greens), shredded

1 tablespoon chopped parsley

1 tablespoon chopped oregano

400g (14oz) can butter beans in water, drained
    and rinsed

Preheat the oven to 190°C (375°F), Gas Mark 5.

Place the aubergine, peppers, red onion, tomatoes, garlic and rosemary sprigs in a roasting tray and drizzle with the olive oil. Roast for 40 minutes, giving them a toss and turn after 20 minutes.

Meanwhile, cook the pasta in a pan of boiling water according to the packet instructions. Drain the pasta, then return to the pan.

When the vegetables are cooked, remove the rosemary and garlic. Now mix the vegetables into the hot pasta and squeeze the garlic cloves out of their skin and into the pasta mix. Tear up the mozzarella and add the chunks to the pasta. Stir well, allowing the mozzarella to melt and the tomatoes to break up.

Add the spinach or other green leaves, herbs and butter beans and stir through, then serve.

> If you double up on the roasted vegetables, you can pop the second batch of veg in the refrigerator or freezer to go with another meal – perfect for when you're in a hurry another day! The roast veg will keep in an airtight container in the refrigerator for up to 3 days and in the freezer for up to 3 months. Reheat in the microwave or in a saucepan before serving (and defrost before reheating, if frozen).

Homemade Falafel Wraps

4 servings (2 portions of veg per serving)

200g (7oz) frozen soybeans (edamame beans),
   or frozen peas, defrosted
400g (14oz) can chickpeas in water, drained
   and rinsed (or use 200g/7oz dried chickpeas,
   soaked and cooked – see Tip)
1 small onion, roughly chopped
2 garlic cloves, crushed
1 teaspoon ground cumin
1 teaspoon ground turmeric

handful of roughly chopped herbs (such
  as coriander)
1 egg, beaten
handful of fresh breadcrumbs (optional)
a little olive oil, for spraying or drizzling

To serve

8 wholemeal tortilla wraps, 2 per person
  (*12 wraps, 3 per person)
hummus (see page 151 for homemade recipe
  or use shop-bought)
mixed salad leaves
Cheesy Courgette Fingers (see page 150)

Preheat the oven to 200°C (400°F), Gas Mark 6. Line a baking tray
with nonstick baking paper.

Place the soybeans or peas, chickpeas, onion, garlic, spices
and herbs in a food processor and whizz to combine. Scrape the
mixture into a bowl, add the egg and mix in by hand. If the mixture
is too wet, add the breadcrumbs so you can shape it into balls.

Shape the falafel mixture into 16 even-sized balls and place
on the lined baking tray. Spray or drizzle with a little olive oil.

Bake for 15–20 minutes or until browned.

Serve 4 falafels per person in wholemeal tortilla wraps with
hummus and salad leaves. Enjoy the cheesy courgette fingers on
the side.

If using dried chickpeas, put them in a bowl and cover with cold water. Leave to soak overnight, then drain and rinse. Put the chickpeas in a saucepan and cover with plenty of fresh water. Bring to the boil, then reduce the heat, cover and simmer for 45–60 minutes or until tender. Drain, cool and use as required.

Simple Pizza

4 servings

olive oil, for greasing
mixed side salad, to serve

For the sauce

400g (14oz) can chopped tomatoes
2 tablespoons tomato purée
1 teaspoon dried mixed herbs or a handful of
    chopped mixed herbs
½ teaspoon caster sugar
freshly ground black pepper

For the pizza base

450g (1lb) plain white flour, plus extra for dusting
150ml (¼ pint) Greek yogurt

Topping ideas

roasted mixed vegetables and torn mozzarella
    (reduced fat, if you choose)
pesto, sliced courgettes, pepper strips, sweetcorn,
    olives and torn mozzarella (reduced fat, if you
    choose)

sliced mushrooms, tomato slices, roasted pepper
strips, sliced chorizo and torn mozzarella
(reduced fat, if you choose)

Preheat the oven to 200°C (400°F), Gas Mark 6. Lightly grease a baking tray with olive oil.

Mix all the sauce ingredients in a small saucepan, bring to the boil, then reduce the heat and simmer for 10 minutes, until thickened and reduced slightly. Remove from the heat.

For the pizza base, place the flour in a large bowl. Mix in the yogurt, then gradually add 100–150ml (3½fl oz–¼ pint) water, a little at a time, until it forms a soft dough.

Tip the dough on to a lightly floured work surface, then roll out until it is 1cm (½ inch) thick. Transfer to the greased baking tray. Spread the tomato sauce evenly over the base, then top with the toppings of your choice.

Bake for 20 minutes or until the dough is slightly browned, the cheese melted and the veg softened.

Serve hot with a side salad.

Any leftovers will keep in an airtight container in the refrigerator for 1 day. Leftover cold pizza will make a tasty lunch for the next day.

Lentil Bolognese

4 servings (3 portions of veg per serving)

1 onion, roughly chopped
3 large peppers (any colour; a great way to use

up the green ones), cored, deseeded and
   cut into chunks
3 large carrots, peeled and cut into chunks
1 broccoli stalk, cut into chunks (see Tip)
½ head of celery, cut into chunks
2 handfuls of green leaves (such as kale, spring
   greens, chard or spinach), shredded
2 garlic cloves, chopped
handful of chopped mixed herbs (such as parsley,
   thyme and oregano)
1 tablespoon olive oil
1 teaspoon ground turmeric
1 teaspoon ground cumin
1 teaspoon ground coriander
400g (14oz) can chopped tomatoes
200g (7oz) dried red lentils
1 tablespoon tomato purée
1 low-salt vegetable stock cube
dried wholewheat pasta of your choice
   (50g/1¾oz, 70g/2½oz or 100g/3½oz per person
   on 1,600/2,000/2,500kcal meal plan)
50g (1¾oz) Cheddar cheese (reduced fat, if you
   choose), grated

Place all the chopped veggies in a food processor, with the green leaves, garlic and herbs, and process to chop finely. You may need to work in a couple of batches. If you prefer, you can finely chop the vegetables by hand.

Heat the olive oil in a saucepan over a medium heat. Add the chopped veg mixture and the ground spices and sauté for about 5 minutes or until softened. Add the canned tomatoes, then fill the can with water and add that to the pan too.

Now add in the lentils and tomato purée, then crumble in the stock cube.

Bring to the boil, then reduce the heat and simmer, uncovered, for about 30 minutes or until thickened, with a similar consistency to Bolognese sauce. Stir the mixture occasionally and top up with a little more water if it is getting too thick.

Meanwhile, cook the pasta in a pan of boiling water according to the packet instructions until al dente, then drain.

Serve the lentil Bolognese with the cooked pasta, with the grated cheese sprinkled over the top.

This is a fabulous recipe to use up any leftover veggies or those bits lurking in the bottom of the refrigerator. I specifically save my broccoli stalks for recipes like this.

Sweet Potato & Kidney Bean Chilli

4 servings (3 portions of veg per serving)

2 sweet potatoes (about 300g/10½oz total weight), peeled and cut into chunks

2 large carrots, peeled and cut into chunks

1 parsnip, peeled and cut into chunks

3 peppers (any colour), cored, deseeded and cut into chunks

1 teaspoon smoked paprika

1 teaspoon ground cumin

1 teaspoon medium chilli powder

1 teaspoon ground cinnamon

1 teaspoon ground ginger

1 teaspoon dried oregano
1 tablespoon olive oil, plus an extra splash
2 garlic cloves, left whole with skin on
brown basmati or brown long-grain rice
  (50g/1¾oz, 70g/2½oz or 100g/3½oz per person
  on 1,600/2,000/2,500kcal meal plan)
1 red onion, chopped
400g (14oz) can chopped tomatoes
400g (14oz) can red kidney beans in water,
  drained and rinsed

Preheat the oven to 200°C (400°F), Gas Mark 6.

Place all the veg chunks in a roasting tin. Sprinkle over the ground spices and dried oregano and stir to coat the chunks, then drizzle over the 1 tablespoon of olive oil and toss gently to mix. Throw in the garlic cloves.

Roast for 40 minutes or until browned at the edges and softened, turning them once halfway through.

When the roast veggies are nearly ready, cook the rice in a pan of boiling water according to the packet instructions until tender, then drain and keep hot.

Heat the remaining splash of olive oil in a large pan over a medium–low heat, then add the red onion and cook gently for 2 minutes. Increase the heat to medium, then add the roast veggies from the oven and squeeze the garlic cloves out of their skin into the pan. Cook for a few minutes, then add the canned tomatoes. Fill the can with water and add that to the pan too. Stir in the kidney beans, then bring to a simmer and cook, uncovered, for 15 minutes or until the consistency has thickened, stirring occasionally.

Serve the chilli with the cooked rice.

Fish & Vegetable Pearl Barley Risotto

4 servings (2 portions of veg per serving)

1 tablespoon olive oil

1 leek, trimmed, cleaned and chopped

2 garlic cloves, crushed

1 carrot, peeled and diced

1 courgette, trimmed and diced

200g (7oz) mushrooms, trimmed and sliced

pearl barley (50g/1¾oz, 70g/2½oz or 100g/3½oz
  per person on 1,600/2,000/2,500kcal meal plan)

2 garlic cloves, crushed

100ml (3½fl oz) dry white wine

800ml (28fl oz) hot chicken stock

400g (14oz) skinless white fish fillets, such as
  haddock, pollock or bass (these can be frozen,
  defrosted fillets)

handful of chopped mixed herbs (such as parsley
  or chives)

2 tablespoons lemon juice

200g (7oz) baby spinach or shredded spinach
  leaves

25g (⅘oz) Parmesan cheese, finely grated

freshly ground black pepper

Preheat the oven to 180°C (350°F), Gas Mark 4.

Drizzle the olive oil into a wide-based frying pan over a medium heat, and add the leek, garlic, carrot, courgette and mushrooms. Let them all cook gently for 10 minutes until softened.

Add the pearl barley and garlic to the pan and stir around for 2 minutes. Now add the white wine and allow this to sizzle and be absorbed while you stir.

Pour the hot chicken stock into the frying pan all at once, then continue to simmer the risotto gently over a medium–low heat, stirring from time to time, for about 15 minutes until all the stock has been absorbed and the pearl barley is tender.

Meanwhile, place the fish fillets on a baking tray, cover with foil, then bake for 10 minutes or until cooked through. Remove from the oven and set aside, still covered, so they retain their heat.

Flake the fish and add this to the pan along with the herbs, lemon juice and some black pepper. Stir through the spinach, allowing it to wilt in the heat.

Serve sprinkled with the Parmesan.

White Fish Stew

4 servings (3–4 portions of veg per serving)

1 tablespoon olive oil

1 red onion, chopped

1 tablespoon sweet paprika

1 teaspoon ground cumin

1 teaspoon ground coriander

2 large garlic cloves, crushed

3–4 rosemary sprigs, according to
your taste

3 bay leaves

2 carrots, peeled and cut into 3cm (1¼ inch)
chunks

1 small butternut squash (250g/9oz), peeled,
deseeded and chopped into 3cm (1¼ inch)
chunks

2 x 400g (14oz) cans chopped tomatoes

400g (14oz) skinless white fish fillets, such as
   pollock, cod or haddock (these can be frozen,
   defrosted fillets), cut into chunks
400g (14oz) can chickpeas in water, drained
   and rinsed
½ head of broccoli (about 150g/5½oz), broken
   into small florets
200g (7oz) green leaves (such as chard, spinach,
   cabbage, kale), shredded if large leaves, left
   whole if small
wholegrain of your choice, such as couscous,
   brown rice, bulgur wheat or freekeh (50g/1¾oz,
   75g/2¾oz or 100g/3½oz per person on
   1,600/2,000/2,500kcal meal plan)
3 tablespoons chopped chives
freshly ground black pepper

Heat the olive oil in a large, wide-based frying pan or flameproof casserole dish over a medium heat. Add the red onion and cook for 5 minutes until softened. Add the ground spices, garlic, rosemary sprigs and bay leaves and cook for 2 minutes.

Now add the carrots and butternut squash, combining them with the spices and herbs. Pour in the canned tomatoes and season with black pepper, then bring to a simmer and cook, covered, for 5–10 minutes or until thickened slightly.

Add the fish fillets, chickpeas and broccoli, pushing them into the sauce, then reduce the heat to medium–low and simmer for 5 minutes, covered, until the fish is cooked and tender. Now stir the green leaves into the stew so they wilt in the heat.

Meanwhile, cook the wholegrain of your choice according to the packet instructions, then drain (if needed). Note, if you are serving brown rice with the stew, then you'll need to start cooking the rice before you start the stew.

Season the stew with black pepper and sprinkle with the chives to garnish. Serve with the cooked wholegrain.

Salmon & Spinach Frittata

4 servings (3 portions of veg per serving)

1 tablespoon olive oil
300g (10½oz) white potatoes, cut into small dice
1 red onion, thinly sliced
8 eggs
handful of mixed herbs (such as parsley, tarragon and thyme), roughly chopped
200g (7oz) skinless salmon fillet, cut into chunks
80g (2¾oz) frozen peas
120g (4¼oz) asparagus tips
½ head of broccoli (about 150g/5½oz), finely chopped
200g (7oz) baby spinach
freshly ground black pepper
mixed side salad, to serve

Heat the olive oil in a wide-based frying pan with a heatproof handle over a medium heat. Add the diced potatoes and cook, stirring occasionally, for about 10 minutes until they are lightly browned and starting to soften. Add the red onion and cook for a further 3 minutes or until softened.

Meanwhile, beat the eggs in a bowl with the herbs and some black pepper. Set aside.

Add the salmon to the pan with a splash of water to prevent it from burning and cook for 3 minutes. Now add the peas, asparagus and broccoli, along with another splash of water, and let it all sauté for 2 minutes.

Arrange the salmon and vegetables evenly over the base of the pan, then pour over the beaten egg mixture. Pop the spinach on top in an even layer, pushing it down under the egg with a wooden spoon. Allow the frittata to cook over a medium–low heat for 10 minutes or until the bottom is cooked and the top is starting to firm a little.

Meanwhile, preheat the grill to medium.

Place the frying pan under the hot grill until the top of the frittata is cooked, about 5 minutes.

Serve immediately with a side salad.

Herb-topped Salmon with Roasted Veggies

4 servings (2 portions of veg per serving)

1 large courgette, trimmed and cut into chunks

1 aubergine (about 250g/9oz), cut into chunks

1 red onion, cut into chunks

2 red, orange or yellow peppers, cored, deseeded and cut into chunks

1 fennel bulb, trimmed and quartered

3 tablespoons olive oil

4 salmon fillets (each about 100g/3½oz)

large handful of chopped mixed herbs (such as chives, parsley and tarragon)

1 slice of wholemeal bread, made into breadcrumbs

1 garlic clove, crushed
wholegrain of your choice, such as couscous,
    bulgur wheat, brown rice or freekeh (50g/1¾oz,
    75g/2¾oz or 100g/3½oz per person on
    1,600/2,000/2,500kcal meal plan)

Preheat the oven to 200°C (400°F), Gas Mark 6. Line a baking tray with nonstick baking paper.

Place all the vegetable chunks in a roasting tray with the fennel quarters. Drizzle with 1 tablespoon of the olive oil and toss to mix. Roast for 15 minutes until softened and charred in places.

Place the salmon fillets in a single layer on the lined baking tray, skin-side down.

Mix the herbs with the breadcrumbs, garlic and the remaining 2 tablespoons of olive oil. Use this mixture to top the salmon fillets – you will need to divide and shape it with your hands to keep it on top of the salmon, pressing it down gently.

Once the vegetables have been roasting for 15 minutes, place the salmon in the oven alongside them and roast for a further 15 minutes until the salmon looks crusty and crunchy on top, and the veg is well cooked and soft to the touch.

Meanwhile, cook the wholegrain of your choice according to the packet instructions, then drain (if needed). Note, if you are serving brown rice with the salmon, then you'll need to start cooking the rice just as you start roasting the veg.

Serve the roast salmon and vegetables immediately with the cooked wholegrain.

Prawn Jackets

4 servings (2 portions of veg per serving)

4 baked potatoes (each the size of your fist,
   or about 200g/7oz)
4 corn on the cob
400g (14oz) frozen raw peeled prawns, defrosted
2 tablespoons low-fat mayonnaise
2 tablespoons Greek yogurt
a pinch of sweet paprika
½ teaspoon tomato purée
reduced-fat olive oil spread
Red Cabbage Slaw (see page 150), to serve

For the salad

200g (7oz) mixed salad leaves
250g (9oz) cherry tomatoes, halved
½ cucumber, sliced
a glug of olive oil
a glug of balsamic vinegar

Preheat the oven to 200°C (400°F), Gas Mark 6.

Wash and prick the potatoes all over, then cook in the microwave on high for 12 minutes. Transfer the potatoes to the oven, placing them directly on the shelf, and cook for a further 30 minutes, until tender. Alternatively, cook them entirely in the oven for 1–1½ hours.

With 10 minutes to go, wrap the corn cobs individually in foil and put on the shelf in the oven alongside the potatoes.

Meanwhile, mix the prawns with the mayo, Greek yogurt, paprika and tomato purée in a bowl, then set aside.

Make the salad. Combine the salad leaves, cherry tomatoes and cucumber in a serving bowl. In a small bowl, whisk together the olive oil and balsamic vinegar, then drizzle over the salad and toss to mix.

Remove the potatoes from the oven, place each one on a serving plate and cut it open. Top each potato with a little reduced-fat spread, then spoon over the prawn mixture.

Serve with the mixed salad and red cabbage slaw.

Fajitas

4 servings (3 portions of veg per serving)

For the fajita seasoning

2 teaspoons smoked paprika
1 teaspoon dried oregano
1 teaspoon ground cumin
1 teaspoon mild chilli powder (optional)

For the fajitas

1 tablespoon olive oil
1 onion, thinly sliced
2 garlic cloves, crushed
400g (14oz) protein (such as thinly sliced raw chicken, beef or firm tofu, or canned beans, drained and rinsed)
2 red, orange or yellow peppers, cored, deseeded and thinly sliced
1 carrot, peeled and thinly sliced
160g (5¾oz) mushrooms, thinly sliced

160g (5¾oz) mangetout (left whole) or green
   beans (trimmed and sliced)
100g (3½oz) tomatoes, chopped
200g (7oz) green leaves (such as spinach,
   Swiss chard or kale), chopped

For the guacamole

flesh from 2 ripe avocados
juice of 1 lime
1 teaspoon lazy garlic (pre-prepped finely
   chopped garlic) or asafoetida

To serve

8 wholemeal tortilla wraps, 2 per person
   (*12 wraps, 3 per person)
150ml (¼ pint) Greek yogurt
80g (2¾oz) Parmesan cheese, grated

Combine all the ingredients for the fajita seasoning mix and set them aside.

For the fajitas, heat the olive oil in a wok over a high heat, then add the onion and stir-fry for 3 minutes. Reduce the heat to medium, add the garlic and stir-fry for 1 minute.

Next, add the protein and stir-fry (for 5 minutes if you're using meat, or 3 minutes if you're using tofu or beans). Add a splash of water, if needed, to prevent it from burning.

Add the peppers, carrot, mushrooms and mangetout or green beans, along with the fajita seasoning mix. Stir-fry for a few minutes, then add the chopped tomatoes. Reduce the heat to medium–low and allow the mixture to simmer for 5 minutes until everything is cooked through.

Meanwhile, make the guacamole. Mash the avocado flesh in a bowl, then stir in the lime juice and lazy garlic or asafoetida.

Remove the wok from the heat. Add the green leaves at the end so they wilt in the residual heat of the wok.

Warm the tortilla wraps in the microwave for 30 seconds. Serve the hot fajita mix with the warmed tortilla wraps, guacamole, Greek yogurt and grated cheese, letting everyone make their own. Tuck in and enjoy.

Green Thai Curry

4 servings (3 portions of veg per serving)

brown basmati or brown long-grain rice
(50g/1¾oz, 70g/2½oz or 100g/3½oz per person
on 1,600/2,000/2,500kcal meal plan)

400g (14oz) skinless chicken thigh fillets or firm
tofu (drained), cut into thin strips

200g (7oz) green beans, trimmed and cut
into strips

1 head of broccoli (about 350g/12oz), broken into
small florets

200g (7oz) baby corn, cut lengthways into strips

2 peppers (any colour), cored, deseeded and cut
into strips

250ml (9fl oz) canned reduced-fat coconut milk
(freeze the rest – see Tips)

large handful of prepared green leaves (such as
baby spinach, shredded chard or spring greens,
or chopped kale)

For the green curry paste

3 green chillies, chopped (deseeded if you prefer
  less heat)
2 shallots, chopped
2 garlic cloves, peeled but left whole
1 lemon grass stalk, trimmed and roughly
  chopped
large handful of fresh coriander, leaves and stalks

Cook the rice in a pan of boiling water according to the packet instructions until tender, then drain.

Meanwhile, make the curry. Make the green curry paste by whizzing all the ingredients together in a food processor to form a paste. Whatever you don't use, pop in the freezer for next time (see Tips).

Add 1–2 tablespoons of the curry paste to a wide-based saucepan over a medium–low heat and cook for 3 minutes until fragrant. Increase the heat to medium, then add the chicken or tofu to the pan and coat in the curry paste. Add the green beans, broccoli, baby corn and peppers and stir well. Cook, stirring regularly, for 5 minutes or until the vegetables are soft.

Add the coconut milk, stir in the green leaves and simmer for 5 minutes until the chicken (if using) is cooked through (when you cut a piece in half, it will be white in the centre).

Serve the curry with the cooked rice.

The leftover curry paste will keep in an airtight container in the refrigerator for up to 4 weeks, or in the freezer for up to 3 months (defrost before use). The leftover coconut milk will keep in an airtight container in the freezer for up to 3 months (defrost before use).

Easy Pad Thai

4 servings (3 portions of veg per serving)

dried brown rice noodles (50g/1¾oz, 70g/2½oz or 100g/3½oz per person on 1,600/2,000/2,500kcal meal plan)

2 teaspoons tamarind paste

2 tablespoons fish sauce

2 teaspoons soft light brown sugar

2 garlic cloves, crushed

juice of 1 lime

1 tablespoon rapeseed oil

1 large carrot, peeled and thinly sliced

1 red pepper, cored, deseeded and thinly sliced

200g (7oz) green beans, trimmed and thinly sliced

6 spring onions, thinly sliced

1 egg

400g (14oz) cold cooked (skinless) chicken, cut into strips, or cooked peeled prawns, or firm tofu, drained and diced

80g (2¾oz) bean sprouts

120g (4¼oz) unsalted peanuts, roughly chopped

4 lime wedges, to serve

Place the noodles in a large, heatproof bowl and pour over enough boiling water to cover. Leave to stand for 5–10 minutes until the noodles are soft, then drain well and set aside (keeping them warm).

Meanwhile, mix the tamarind paste, fish sauce, sugar, garlic and lime juice together in a small bowl and set aside.

Heat the rapeseed oil in a wok over a high heat. Once hot, add the carrot, red pepper and green beans and stir-fry for 3 minutes, then add the spring onions. Push the vegetables to one side of the wok, then crack the egg into the centre of the wok. Stir it until it begins to set and resembles a broken-up omelette.

Next, add in the protein (cooked chicken, prawns or tofu) along with the tamarind mixture. Give it all a good mix and stir-fry for 3 minutes, until the protein has a light brown colour.

Add the bean sprouts and warm noodles and toss together well.

Serve immediately, scattered with the chopped peanuts, with a lime wedge (for squeezing) to accompany each portion.

Chicken Curry

4 servings (2–3 portions of veg per serving)

brown basmati or brown long-grain rice
 (50g/1¾oz, 70g/2½oz or 100g/3½oz per person
 on 1,600/2,000/2,500kcal meal plan)
1 tablespoon rapeseed oil
1 teaspoon mustard seeds
1 tablespoon ground cumin
1 tablespoon ground coriander
½ tablespoon ground turmeric
5mm (¼ inch) piece of fresh root ginger, grated
 or 1 tablespoon ground ginger

300g (10½oz) boneless, skinless chicken breast
fillets, cut into bitesize chunks

400g (14oz) can chopped tomatoes

400g (14oz) can brown or green lentils in water,
drained and rinsed, or 150g (5½oz) dried split
red lentils

2 carrots, peeled diced

1 small swede or 1 large parsnip, peeled and diced,
or 250g (9oz) butternut squash, peeled,
deseeded and diced

½ cauliflower (about 300g/10½oz), broken into
small florets

1 green pepper, cored, deseeded and diced

1 tablespoon tomato purée

Cook the rice in a pan of boiling water according to the packet instructions until tender, then drain.

Meanwhile, make the curry. Heat the rapeseed oil in a wide-based saucepan over a high heat until hot. Add in all the spices, reduce the heat to low and cook for 2 minutes until fragrant. Add the ginger and chicken and cook over a medium heat until the chicken is browned all over, about 5 minutes.

Pour in the canned tomatoes and lentils and bring to a simmer. Next, add all the vegetables, tomato purée and 100ml (3½fl oz) water (rinsing out the tomato can with the measured water, if you like). Bring to the boil, then reduce the heat and simmer with the lid on, stirring occasionally, for 15 minutes, or until the lentils are cooked and the sauce has thickened.

Serve the chicken curry with the cooked brown rice.

Sweet & Sour Pork

4 servings (3 portions of veg per serving)

brown basmati or brown long-grain rice
(50g/1¾oz, 70g/2½oz or 100g/3½oz per person
on 1,600/2,000/2,500kcal meal plan)

2 tablespoons olive oil

400g (14oz) lean pork fillet, cut into bite-sized
pieces

1 garlic clove, crushed

2 carrots, peeled and thinly sliced into strips

1 red pepper, cored, deseeded and sliced
into strips

2 yellow peppers, cored, deseeded and sliced
into strips

8 celery sticks, roughly chopped

8 spring onions, chopped into 4 cm (1½ inch)
lengths

160g (5¾oz) mangetout (left whole) or green
beans (trimmed and halved)

160g (5¾oz) baby corn, halved lengthways

4 canned pineapple slices in fruit juice, drained
and chopped

For the sweet and sour sauce

2 tablespoons reduced-salt soy sauce

1 tablespoon low-salt, low-sugar tomato ketchup

2 tablespoons rice vinegar or dry sherry

Cook the rice in a pan of boiling water according to the packet
instructions until tender, then drain.

Meanwhile, make the stir-fry. First, make the sweet and sour sauce by mixing together the soy sauce, tomato ketchup and vinegar or sherry in a small bowl. Set aside.

Next, heat the olive oil in a wok over a high heat. Once hot, add the pork and stir-fry for 5 minutes until it is cooked and beginning to colour, then transfer to a plate with a slotted spoon and set aside.

Add the garlic, carrots and peppers to the juices left in the wok and stir-fry over a high heat for 3 minutes. Next, add the rest of the vegetables and stir-fry for another few minutes, adding in a splash or two of water, if needed, to stop the veg from sticking.

Return the pork to the wok, along with the pineapple, and pour over the sweet and sour sauce. Reduce the heat and simmer for about 3 minutes until warmed through.

Serve the sweet and sour pork with the cooked brown rice.

Steak with Sweet Potato Fries & Roasted Veggies

4 servings (3 portions of veg per serving)

4 sirloin steaks (each about 150g/5½oz)

4 teaspoons olive oil, plus an extra drizzle

1 courgette, trimmed and cut into chunks

1 red pepper, cored, deseeded and cut into chunks

1 yellow pepper, cored, deseeded and cut into chunks

1 aubergine (about 350g/12oz), cut into chunks

4 portobello mushrooms or 12 small mushrooms, left whole

2 large sweet potatoes (about 400g/14oz in total), scrubbed

1 teaspoon smoked paprika
1 teaspoon dried oregano
freshly ground black pepper
mustard of your choice, to serve

Preheat the oven to 220°C (425°F), Gas Mark 7.

Place the steaks on a large plate and drizzle with olive oil. Rub in the oil, then cover and allow them to come to room temperature.

Meanwhile, place the courgette, pepper and aubergine chunks in a roasting tin. Drizzle over 2 teaspoons of the olive oil and toss to mix. Roast for 30–40 minutes, turning them over halfway through cooking. Add the mushrooms to the roasting tin for the final 15 minutes of the cooking time.

Meanwhile, cut the sweet potatoes into fries (each about the size of your index finger). Place in a mixing bowl and toss with the remaining 2 teaspoons of olive oil, along with the paprika and dried oregano. Spread out in a single layer on a large nonstick baking tray and roast alongside the veggies for 30 minutes or until crispy. Turn the fries or give the tray a good shake halfway through cooking.

While the veggies and fries finish roasting, heat a nonstick frying pan or ridged griddle pan over a high heat. Once hot, place the steaks in the pan (there is no need to oil the pan as there will still be oil on the steaks from earlier) and cook for 2–3 minutes without moving them. Then turn them over and cook for a few minutes on the other side. Look for the change in colour as the steaks cook: when the colour-change reaches about halfway up, then you know to turn them). Cook the steaks to your liking.

Transfer the cooked steaks to a warm plate. Cover them loosely with foil and leave to rest and stay warm while you serve up.

Divide the roasted veggies and fries between serving plates, then serve the steaks alongside. Serve with a good dollop of mustard and plenty of black pepper.

Snacks, Sides & Sweet Nibbles

Red Cabbage Slaw

4 servings (2 portions of veg per serving)

300g (10½oz) red cabbage, finely shredded
1 large carrot, peeled and grated
1 large dessert apple, peeled, cored and grated
bunch of spring onions, thinly sliced
handful of chives, chopped
50g (1¾oz) raisins
2 tablespoons red wine vinegar
1 tablespoon low-fat mayonnaise
freshly ground black pepper

You can either shred/grate the cabbage, carrot and apple by hand or using a food processor.

Place the cabbage, carrot, apple, spring onions and chives in a large bowl and mix well. Add the raisins, then stir in the vinegar and mayo until combined. Season with black pepper.

Serve, or cover and keep in the refrigerator for up to 3 days.

Cheesy Courgette Fingers

4 servings (1 portion of veg per serving)

2 courgettes, trimmed
2 tablespoons plain white or wholemeal flour
1 egg, beaten
3 tablespoons fine cornmeal or polenta
50g (1¾oz) Cheddar cheese (reduced fat, if you choose), grated

Preheat the oven to 200°C (400°F), Gas Mark 6. Line a baking tray with nonstick baking paper.

Cut the courgettes into fingers, each about the thickness and length of your thumb.

Put the flour into one bowl, the beaten egg into another and the cornmeal mixed with the cheese into a third bowl.

Dip each courgette finger first into the flour, then the egg, then the cornmeal/cheese mixture to coat, then place on the lined baking tray. Repeat until all the courgette fingers are coated.

Bake for 20 minutes until crispy and a little brown. These are best served hot, straight from the oven.

Hummus

6–8 servings

400g (14oz) can chickpeas in water, drained and rinsed
1 garlic clove, roughly chopped
1 tablespoon tahini
juice of 1 lemon
3 tablespoons olive oil
3 tablespoons natural yogurt

Place the chickpeas, garlic, tahini and lemon juice in a food processor. Start to blend and slowly drizzle in the olive oil as you go (with the processor running). Add the yogurt and whizz to a smooth consistency.

Scrape into a bowl and serve immediately, or store in an airtight container in the refrigerator for up to 3 days.

Spiced Roasted Chickpeas

8–14 servings (1 serving = 28g (1oz) or
  ### *50g/1¾oz)

½ teaspoon mild chilli powder
½ teaspoon ground coriander
½ teaspoon ground cumin
½ teaspoon ground turmeric
½ teaspoon asafoetida
1 tablespoon rapeseed oil, plus extra for greasing
400g (14oz) can chickpeas in water, drained and
  rinsed (or use 200g/7oz dried chickpeas,
  soaked overnight and cooked until soft –
  see Tip on page 125)

Preheat the oven to 200°C (400°F), Gas Mark 6.

Mix the ground spices in a bowl with the rapeseed oil, then add in the chickpeas and toss to coat them in the spice mixture. Tip on to a greased baking tray and spread out into a single layer.

Roast for 30 minutes or until crispy, shaking the tray halfway through to make sure they don't stick.

Remove from the oven and leave to cool completely on the tray, then transfer to an airtight container – they will keep for up to 7 days.

Energy Balls

Makes 10 balls (a serving is 1–2 balls) (½ portion
  ### of fruit/veg per ball)

150g (5½oz) dried pitted dates
150g (5½oz) ready-to-eat dried apricots

150g (5½oz) rolled oats
75g (2¾oz) almonds
75g (2¾oz) walnuts
1 carrot, peeled and finely grated
1 teaspoon ground cinnamon
1 teaspoon ground ginger
1 teaspoon ground mixed spice

Place the dates, apricots and oats into a food processor. Whizz together to make a paste, adding a splash of water if needed.
Add the almonds and walnuts and process these too until finely chopped. (If you prefer, you can scrape out the dried fruit paste into a bowl, then process the nuts separately until finely chopped).

Scrape the mixture into a bowl, add the grated carrot and ground spices and mix well.

Take 2 teaspoons of the mixture and roll it into a ball, then place on a plate. Repeat with the remaining mixture to make a total of 10 balls. Store the energy balls in an airtight container in the refrigerator for up to 3 days, or in the freezer for up to 3 months.

Banana Flapjacks

12 servings (½ portion of fruit per serving)

2 large ripe bananas, peeled
250g (9oz) rolled oats
100g (3½oz) raisins
40g (1½oz) sesame seeds
40g (1½oz) pumpkin seeds
150g (5½oz) reduced-fat olive oil spread,
   plus extra for greasing
2 tablespoons thick or clear honey

Preheat the oven to 180°C (350°F), Gas Mark 4. Grease and line a 20cm (8 inch) square shallow baking tin.

Mash the bananas in a heatproof bowl, then stir in the oats, raisins and seeds.

Place the olive-oil spread and honey in a suitable bowl and heat in the microwave on medium for 1 minute at a time until melted together (or you can do this in a small saucepan over a low heat).

Pour the melted butter mixture into the banana-and-oat mixture and mix well to combine. Tip into the prepared tin and spread it out evenly.

Bake for 45 minutes until lightly browned on the top and firm. About halfway through the baking time, I suggest covering the top with foil or greaseproof paper to prevent the seeds and raisins from burning.

Remove from the oven and cool slightly, then mark into 12 squares. Transfer to a wire rack and leave to cool completely in the tin.

Once cold, cut into squares, remove from the tin and serve. Store in an airtight container for up to 3 days. These flapjacks also freeze well for up to 3 months (defrost at room temperature before serving).

Fruity Crumble

6 servings (1 portion of fruit per serving)

500g (1lb 2oz) prepared (peeled, cored and chopped/sliced) fruit (frozen, defrosted fruit works well to save time, or use a combination of whatever needs using up in the fruit bowl!)

200g (7oz) rolled oats

50g (1¾oz) ground almonds
75g (2¾oz) reduced-fat olive oil spread
75g (2¾oz) soft light brown sugar
2 teaspoons ground cinnamon
1 teaspoon ground mixed spice

Preheat the oven to 200°C (400°F), Gas Mark 6.

If using fresh fruit, place it in a pan with a couple of tablespoons of water. Cook over a gentle heat for about 5 minutes until it softens. Remove from the heat.

Place the softened fresh fruit or defrosted frozen fruit into an ovenproof dish.

In a bowl, mix together the oats, ground almonds, reduced-fat spread, sugar, cinnamon and mixed spice, lightly rubbing the margarine into the dry ingredients as you mix until you have a crumbly mixture.

Spoon the oat mixture on top of the fruit in an even layer, covering it completely.

Bake for 30 minutes or until browned on the top. Serve hot, warm or cold.

Banana 'Ice Cream'

1 serving (1 portion of fruit per serving)

1 ripe banana, peeled and cut into chunks
½ teaspoon ground cinnamon or unsweetened
   cocoa powder

Place the banana chunks in a small, freezerproof container and freeze until firm, about 1–2 hours.

Transfer the frozen chunks into a small food processor, add the cinnamon or cocoa powder and whizz together to combine.

Scrape into a bowl and serve immediately.

Frozen Raspberry or Mango Fool

2 servings (2 portions of fruit per serving)

2 handfuls of frozen raspberries or frozen mango chunks (about 250g/9oz)
1 ripe banana, peeled
4 tablespoons natural yogurt

Place the frozen raspberries or mango in a small food processor with the banana and yogurt. Whizz together until combined.

Transfer to two serving glasses or small dishes and serve immediately.

Quick Baked Apple

1 serving (1 portion of fruit per serving)

1 dessert apple, cored
2 teaspoons dried fruit (such as raisins or chopped apricots)
sprinkle of ground cinnamon
1 tablespoon unsweetened apple juice or water
natural yogurt, to serve

Place the apple in a microwave-safe bowl. Fill the centre of the apple with the dried fruit, sprinkle over the cinnamon, then pour the apple juice or water around it in the bowl.

Microwave on high for about 2 minutes, then check to see if it's cooked and softened. If not, microwave for another 30 seconds or until cooked.

Remove from the microwave and leave to stand for a couple of minutes, then serve with yogurt.

To make this recipe using a regular oven, preheat the oven to 200°C (400°F), Gas Mark 6. Place the prepared apple on a baking tray and cook for 20 minutes.

7

Meal Plans & Shopping Lists

These meal plans are not here to be prescriptive, but to give you a guide: to show how you can fit all the foods into your day and how to get variety across the week. Once you get into the habit of meal planning, you will find it becomes second nature to include all your portions per day and to have that balance.

The meal plans are designed to feed a single person, with the exception of dinner, which consists of 4 servings. The plans are based on 2,000kcals, so if you are on the 1,600kcal meal plan, then you will only need one snack instead of two. However, if you are hungry, then do respond to that signal, as we are not being calorie precise here. You could also spread lunch out by saving an item from that meal for your afternoon snack. You will see asterisks (*) alongside some of the ingredient measurements (in brackets). These are larger portion sizes for those following the 2,500kcal meal plan.

We've provided a shopping list for each week of the plan. As long as your storecupboard is also well-stocked (see pages 161–3), you will have all you need to follow the meal plan if you buy everything on the shopping list each week.

Top tips

- Save your broccoli stalks for a stir-fry/lentil Bolognese.
- Grow your own herbs and spinach or other greens (such as Swiss chard, kale, collard greens and even beetroot – you can eat the leaves). It can be so easy.
- Use frozen veggies, as this saves time and money. For example, frozen peas and spinach are so useful, and it means you don't have to rely on always having fresh vegetables in for a dish.
- Make full use of your freezer – freeze all your odds and ends for another meal. Or, if you are buying a large amount of something, freeze whatever you do not need. This works with items including ham and other meats, bread products, coconut milk and curry paste.
- Make friends with your local greengrocer. They often have reduced-price produce that will need using that day, which can save you pennies and provide inspiration. The greengrocer's is also a great place to find more unusual fruit and vegetables – plus, buying your food there helps you to eat in season.
- Join a veg box scheme if you cannot get to the greengrocer regularly.
- Keep a supply of frozen fruit for use in breakfasts, smoothies and desserts.
- If you have lots of vegetables that need using up, cook a vegetable side dish, such as a vegetable curry or a tray of roasted veg, and freeze it for another day.
- If you do not have fresh lemons, lemon juice in a squeeze bottle is a good substitute.

Your storecupboard

Dried herbs & spices

asafoetida

black pepper

chilli powder

dried bay leaves

dried mixed herbs

dried oregano

ground cinnamon

ground coriander

ground cumin

ground ginger

ground mixed spice

ground turmeric

mustard seeds

smoked paprika

sweet paprika

Oils & vinegars

balsamic vinegar

cider vinegar

lemon juice

olive oil

rapeseed oil

red wine vinegar

rice vinegar

Dried fruit, nuts & seeds

chia seeds

dried fruit (such as apricots, dates, raisins)

flaxseeds (linseeds)

nuts (unsalted peanuts, almonds, walnuts, cashew nuts)

pumpkin seeds

sesame seeds

Wholegrains

brown basmati or brown long-grain rice
bulgur wheat
couscous
dried brown rice noodles
dried chickpeas
dried split red lentils
oatcakes

rolled oats
wholegrain breadsticks
wholegrain cereal (wheat bisks)
wholegrain crackers
wholewheat pasta

Spreads, sauces & condiments

bottled lemon juice
chutney (tomato, onion or your particular favourite)
Dijon mustard
fish sauce
honey (thick or clear)
maple syrup
mayonnaise (low fat)

peanut butter (low salt and sugar)
soy sauce (reduced salt)
tahini
tomato ketchup (low salt and sugar)
tomato purée
yeast extract

Refrigerator & freezer

reduced-fat olive oil spread
fresh root ginger (keep this in the freezer and grate it from frozen as you need it)
frozen soybeans (edamame beans)

frozen mixed berries
frozen peas
frozen spinach
frozen sweetcorn kernels

Miscellaneous

baking powder

bicarbonate of soda

canned chopped tomatoes

canned reduced-fat coconut
  milk

caster sugar

chicken stock cubes
  (low salt)

cornflour

cornmeal/polenta

garlic (fresh, 'lazy' and
  granules)

gravy granules (low salt)

ground almonds

plain white flour

plain wholemeal flour

roasted peppers in a jar

soft light brown sugar

tamarind paste

vegetable stock cubes
  (low salt)

WEEK 1

	Breakfast	Snack	Lunch
Prepare ahead		Energy Balls (see page 152)	Quick Tuna Pasta Salad (see page 118) Chicken & Bean Salad (see page 119)
Mon	2 slices (*3 slices) of wholemeal toast with peanut butter and slices of banana	Apple and 25g/⅘oz (*30g/1oz) nuts	Quick Tuna Pasta Salad (see page 118); 100ml (3½fl oz) yogurt
Tues	Wholegrain cereal (wheat bisks) with semi-skimmed or skimmed milk and banana	Handful of berries with 100ml (3½fl oz) yogurt (*and 25g/⅘oz seeds)	Quick Tuna Pasta Salad (see page 118); 100ml (3½fl oz) yogurt
Wed	Smoked Salmon Bagel (see page 106); a glass of semi-skimmed or skimmed milk	Latte with skimmed milk; a pear (*and 25g/⅘oz nuts)	Hummus & Veggie Sandwich (see page 112); 25g/⅘oz (*30g/1oz) nuts; a piece of fruit
Thurs	Overnight Oats with Mixed Berries (see page 98)	Carrot sticks and 1 tbsp cream cheese	Chicken & Bean Salad (see page 119); 100ml (3½fl oz) yogurt
Fri	Porridge with Apple & Cinnamon (see page 100)	3 dried apricots (*4) and 25g/⅘oz (*30g/1oz) nuts	Chicken & Bean Salad (see page 119); 100ml (3½fl oz) yogurt
Sat	Banana & Pumpkin Seed Pancakes (see page 101)	Smoothie made with 100ml (3½fl oz) semi-skimmed or skimmed milk and a handful of frozen fruit, plus ½ teaspoon honey if needed	One Pan All-day Veggie Brunch (see page 115)
Sun	BLTM (see page 106); a milky drink (made with semi-skimmed or skimmed milk) or yogurt	Energy Balls (see page 152) x 2 (*3)	White Bean and Pepper Nachos (see page 111)

* extras for the 2,500kcal plan

Snack	Dinner	Dessert
Hummus (see page 151) Banana Flapjacks (see page 153)	Homemade falafels (see page 123)	
Hummus (see page 151) and vegetable sticks (*3 oatcakes)	Sweet & Sour Pork (see page 144)	Fruit and 100ml (3½fl oz) yogurt
Red pepper strips and 1 tablespoon Spiced Roasted Chickpeas (see page 152)	Homemade Falafel Wraps (see page 123)	Frozen Raspberry Fool (see page 156)
1 x Banana Flapjack (see page 153) (*2 flapjacks); a banana	White Fish Stew (see page 131)	Fruit and 100ml (3½fl oz) yogurt
2 small oranges (*and 25g/⅘oz nuts)	Roasted Veggie Pasta (see page 122)	1 x Banana Flapjack (see page 153) (*2 flapjacks); a banana
Fruit and 100ml (3½fl oz) yogurt	Chicken Curry (see page 142)	Melon and berries
40g (1½oz) Cheddar cheese (reduced fat, if you choose) with carrot sticks and cucumber (*3 oatcakes)	Easy Pad Thai (see page 141)	Banana 'Ice Cream' (see page 155) (*and 25g/⅘oz nuts)
Fruit and 100ml (3½fl oz) yogurt	Salmon & Spinach Frittata (see page 133)	Fruity Crumble (see page 154) with custard

WEEK 1 SHOPPING LIST

Fruit and veg

120g (4¼oz) asparagus tips

1 aubergine

1 avocado

160g (5¾oz) baby corn

2 x 200g (7oz) bags baby spinach

8 bananas

80g (2¾oz) bean sprouts

1 broccoli

1 butternut squash

10 carrots

1 cauliflower

1 celery

1 x 250g (9oz) punnet cherry tomatoes

3 courgettes

1 small cucumber

2 dessert apples

fresh herbs, including chives, oregano, parsley and rosemary

1 x 500g (1lb 2oz) bag frozen fruit of your choice

1 garlic bulb

200g (7oz) green beans

80g (2¾oz) frozen peas

1 green pepper

2 lemons

2 limes

160g (5¾oz) mangetout

1 melon

200g (7oz) mixed berries

1 x 1kg (2lb 4oz) bag frozen mixed berries

4 x 120g (4¼oz) bags mixed salad leaves

1 x 200g (7oz) punnet mushrooms

1 small onion

5 red onions

2 small oranges

1 pear

1 x 227g (8oz) can pineapple slices in fruit juice

1 x 350g (12oz) bag frozen raspberries

7 red peppers

2 bunches of spring onions

2 x 198g (7oz) cans salt-free sweetcorn kernels

11 tomatoes

1 x 1.5kg (3lb 5oz) bag white potatoes

4 yellow peppers

Note: If you follow meal plans 1–3 week by week you may find that you have leftover ingredients that can be rolled over to the next week.

Dairy	Grains	Protein
1 x 220g (7¾oz) packet Cheddar cheese (reduced fat, if you choose)	1 x 500g (1lb 2oz) packet fine cornmeal or polenta	16 eggs
1 x 300g (10½oz) pot cottage cheese with chives	1 loaf wholegrain bread	400g (14oz) can brown or green lentils in water
	1 packet wholemeal bagels (freeze the ones you don't use)	400g (14oz) can butter beans in water
1 x 500g (1lb 2oz) carton ready-to-serve custard		4 x 400g (14oz) cans chickpeas in water
1 x 500g (1lb 2oz) carton Greek yogurt	1 packet wholegrain cereal (wheat bisks)	400g (14oz) can mixed beans in water
1 x 150g (5½oz) packet mozzarella (reduced fat, if you choose)	2 packets wholemeal tortilla wraps	400g (14oz) can white beans in water
1 x 1kg (2lb 4oz) carton natural yogurt		400g (14oz) chicken breasts
1 litre semi-skimmed or skimmed milk		400g (14oz) chicken, raw peeled prawns or firm tofu
		400g (14oz) lean pork fillet
		1 small packet rindless unsmoked back bacon rashers or medallions
		4 fresh salmon fillets (400g/14oz in total)
		100g (3½oz) smoked salmon
		145g (5¼oz) can tuna in spring water
		4 white fish fillets, fresh or frozen (400g/14oz in total)

WEEK 2

	Breakfast	Snack	Lunch
Prepare ahead	Carrot Cake Muffins (see page 102)		Hummus (see page 151)
Mon	2 slices of whole-meal toast with Marmite and 2 slices of Cheddar cheese (reduced fat, if you choose); a piece of fruit	Fruit and 100ml (3½fl oz) yogurt with seeds	Salmon & Spinach Frittata (see page 133)
Tues	Smoked Salmon Bagel (see page 106); a glass of semi-skimmed or skimmed milk	Smoothie made with 100ml (3½fl oz) semi-skimmed or skimmed milk and a handful of frozen fruit, plus ½ teaspoon honey if needed	Beany Pitta Pockets (see page 114); a piece of fruit
Wed	Wholegrain cereal (wheat bisks) with semi-skimmed or skimmed milk and berries	A banana spread with nut butter and a few seeds	Beany Pitta Pockets (see page 114); a piece of fruit
Thurs	Carrot Cake Muffins (see page 102); a glass of semi-skimmed or skimmed milk	Energy Balls (left-over from Week 1) (see page 152) x 2 (*3)	Mackerel & Beetroot Salad (see page 117); a handful of Spiced Roasted Chickpeas (see page 152); a piece of fruit
Fri	Overnight Oats with Mixed Berries (see page 98)	Fruit and 100ml (3½fl oz) yogurt (*and 25g/⅘oz nuts)	Egg Mayo Sandwich (see page 113); fruit and 100ml (3½fl oz) yogurt
Sat	100ml (3½fl oz) Greek yogurt with fruit and 20g/¾oz (*25g/⅘oz) seeds	Latte with skimmed milk; an apple	2 eggs, scrambled and ½ x 400g (14oz) can low-salt/sugar baked beans on 2 x slices of wholemeal toast with cooked tomatoes
Sun	Tropical Fruit Cup (see page 98)	Apple and 25g/⅘oz (*30g/1oz) nuts	Picking platter: oatcakes, Hummus (see page 151), Cheddar cheese (reduced fat, if you choose), a side plate of mixed salad, grapes, chutney

* extras for the 2,500kcal plan

Snack	Dinner	Snack
	Green curry paste (see page 140)	Banana Flapjacks (see page 153)
Red pepper strips and 1 tablespoon Spiced Roasted Chickpeas (see page 152)	Sweet & Sour Pork (see page 144)	Canned fruit with 100ml (3½fl oz) yogurt
Energy Balls (see page 152) x 2 (*3)	Prawn Jackets (see page 136) with Red Cabbage Slaw (see page 150)	Fruity Crumble (see page 154) with custard (leftover from Sunday)
1 x hard-boiled egg (*2 eggs) with a handful of spinach leaves	Green Thai Curry (see page 139)	40g (1½oz) Cheddar cheese (reduced fat, if you choose) and 3 wholegrain crackers (*5 crackers) with grapes
Hummus (see page 151) and vegetable sticks (*3 oatcakes)	2 chicken sausages (*3) cooked in the oven, with roasted vegetables and brown rice	Fruit salad and 100ml (3½fl oz) yogurt
Hummus (see page 151) and vegetable sticks (*3 oatcakes)	Fish & Vegetable Pearl Barley Risotto (see page 130)	Frozen Mango Fool (see page 156)
3 dried apricots (*4) and 25g/⅞oz (*30g/1oz) nuts	Steak with Sweet Potato Fries & Roasted Veggies (see page 145)	Banana Flapjack (see page 153); a banana
Smoothie made with 100ml (3½fl oz) semi-skimmed or skimmed milk, a banana and a handful of frozen fruit, plus ½ teaspoon honey if needed	Fajitas (see page 137)	100ml (3½fl oz) yogurt with fruit and seeds

WEEK 2 SHOPPING LIST

Fruit and veg

4 apples

120g (4¼oz) asparagus tips

2 aubergines

2 avocados

360g (12½oz) baby corn

3 x 200g (7oz) bags baby spinach

4 baking potatoes

1 beetroot

2 broccoli

1 celery

2 x 250g (9oz) punnets cherry tomatoes

3 courgettes

4 corn cobs

2 cucumbers

7 bananas

9 carrots

1 cooking apple

fresh herbs, including chives, coriander and parsley

1 x 500g (1lb 2oz) bag frozen fruit of your choice

a bunch of grapes

1 x 200g (7oz) pack green beans

3 green chillies

1 x 200g (7oz) bag kale

3 lemons

1 lemon grass stalk

1 leek

1 lime

320g (11½oz) mangetout

1 melon

1 x 500g (1lb 2oz) bag frozen mango

1 x 1kg (2lb 4oz) bag frozen mixed berries

200g (7oz) mixed berries

4 x 120g (4¼oz) bags mixed salad leaves

2 x 200g (7oz) punnets mushrooms

2 nectarines

1 onion

2 orange peppers

2 oranges

2 peaches

2 pears

3 x 227g (8oz) can pineapple slices in fruit juice

4 portobello mushrooms

1 small red cabbage

1 red onion

5 red peppers

2 x 198g (7oz) cans salt-free sweetcorn kernels

2 shallots

2 bunches of spring onions

2 large sweet potatoes

8 tomatoes

1 x 1.5kg (3lb 5oz) bag white potatoes

4 yellow peppers

Note: If you follow meal plans 1–3 week by week you may find that you have leftover ingredients that can be rolled over to the next week.

Dairy	Grains	Protein
1 x 220g (7¾oz) packet Cheddar cheese (reduced fat, if you choose)	1 x 500g (1lb 2oz) packet low-sugar granola	12 eggs
1 x 500g (1lb 2oz) carton ready-to-serve custard	1 x 500g (1lb 2oz) packet pearl barley	2 x 400g (14oz) can butter beans in water
1 x 1kg (2lb 4oz) carton Greek yogurt	1 packet wholemeal bagels (freeze the ones you don't use)	400g (14oz) can low-salt/sugar baked beans 2 x 400g (14oz) can chickpeas in water
1 x 1kg (2lb 4oz) carton natural yogurt	1 loaf wholemeal bread	400g (14oz) chicken, beef, firm tofu or canned beans
1 x 200g (7oz) packet Parmesan cheese	1 packet wholemeal pitta bread (freeze the ones you don't use)	8–10 chicken sausages
1 litre semi-skimmed or skimmed milk	2 packets wholemeal tortilla wraps	400g (14oz) chicken thigh fillet
250g (9oz) soft cheese		400g (14oz) lean pork fillet
		400g (14oz) frozen raw peeled prawns
		2 fresh salmon fillets (200g/7oz in total)
		4 x sirloin steaks (600g/1lb 5oz in total)
		2 x smoked mackerel fillets (250g/9oz in total)
		100g (3½oz) smoked salmon
		4 white fish fillets, fresh or frozen (400g /14oz in total)

Miscellaneous

1 small 187ml (6½fl oz) bottle dry white wine

WEEK 3

	Breakfast	Snack	Lunch
Prepare ahead	Carrot Cake Muffins (see page 102)	Banana Flapjacks (see page 153) Energy Balls (see page 152)	Green Veg Minestrone Soup (see page 110)
Mon	Wholegrain cereal (wheat bisks) with semi-skimmed or skimmed milk and fruit	Latte with skimmed milk; 2 x plain biscuits (*3 biscuits)	Green Veg Minestrone Soup (see page 110) with a wholemeal roll
Tues	1 poached or fried egg and 2 slices of toast (*2 poached or fried eggs and 2 slices of toast) with pan-cooked tomatoes and peppers	2 small oranges and (*25g/⅞oz) nuts	½ x 400g (14oz) can low-salt/low sugar baked beans on 2 x wholemeal toast with 25g (⅞oz) grated Cheddar cheese (reduced fat, if you choose) 1 x yogurt
Wed	Carrot Cake Muffins (see page 102); 100ml (3½fl oz) yogurt	Fruit and 100ml (3½fl oz) yogurt with seeds	Green Veg Minestrone Soup (see page 110) with a wholemeal roll
Thurs	Porridge with Apple & Cinnamon (see page 100)	Energy Balls (see page 152) x 2 (*3)	Lentil Salad (see page 116); fruit and 100ml (3½fl oz) yogurt
Fri	Overnight Oats with Mixed Berries (see page 98)	Banana Flapjack (see page 153); an apple	Ham salad sandwich with 1 slice of ham and a generous portion of salad in 2 slices of wholemeal bread (*3 slices) with mustard and reduced-fat olive oil spread; Hummus (see page 151) with raw vegetables; 100ml (3½fl oz) yogurt
Sat	Banana & Pumpkin Seed Pancakes (see page 101); a milky drink made from semi-skimmed or skimmed milk		Easy Tortilla Pizza (see page 115); 100ml (3½fl oz) yogurt
Sun	Mediterranean Veg Omelette (see page 104); a milky drink made from semi-skimmed or skimmed milk	Latte with skimmed milk; Banana Flapjack (see page 153) or a piece of cake (Madeira, ginger or apple cake)	One Pan All-day Veggie Brunch (see page 115)

* extras for the 2,500kcal plan

Snack	Dinner	Snack
A hard-boiled egg with raw vegetables	Sweet Potato & Kidney Bean Chilli (see page 128)	Fruit and 100ml (3½fl oz) yogurt
Fruit and 100ml (3½fl oz) yogurt	Lentil Bolognese (see page 126)	Smoothie made with 100ml (3½fl oz) semi-skimmed or skimmed milk and a handful of frozen fruit, plus ½ teaspoon honey if needed
Red pepper strips and 1 tablespoon Spiced Roasted Chickpeas (see page 152)	Roasted Veggie Pasta (see page 122)	40g (1½oz) Cheddar cheese (reduced fat, if you choose) and 3 wholegrain crackers (*5 crackers) with grapes
Smoothie made with 100ml (3½fl oz) semi-skimmed or skimmed milk, a banana and a handful of frozen fruit, plus ½ teaspoon honey if needed	Herb-topped Salmon with Roasted Veggies (see page 134)	25g (⅘oz) nuts and 25g (⅘oz) baked crisps with 1 tablespoon Hummus (see page 151)
3 oatcakes (*5 oatcakes), grapes and 40g (1½oz) Cheddar cheese (reduced fat if you choose)	Simple Pizza (see page 125)	Banana 'Ice Cream' (see page 155)
Toasted pitta bread strips, Hummus (see page 151) and raw veggies	Green Thai Curry (see page 139) using curry paste from the freezer	100ml (3½fl oz) yogurt with berries and 20g/¾oz (25g/⅘oz) nuts
3 dried apricots (*4) and 25g/⅘oz (*30g/1oz) nuts	100g (*150g) roast chicken with 2 portions of veg (e.g. broccoli and parsnips), roasted potatoes with skins on and low-salt gravy	Baked Apple (see page 156) with custard

WEEK 3 SHOPPING LIST

Fruit and veg

5 apples

8 bananas

1 bunch asparagus

2 aubergines

200g (7oz) baby corn

3 x 200g (7oz) bags baby spinach

2 broccoli

12 carrots

250g (9oz) punnet cherry tomatoes

1 celery

2 courgettes

1 cucumber

fresh herbs, including mint, oregano, parsley and rosemary

1 fennel bulb

a bunch of grapes

200g (7oz) green beans

1 x 200g (7oz) bag green leaves (spinach, spring greens kale or chard)

4 green peppers

1 lemon

1 x 1kg (2lb 4oz) bag frozen mixed berries

200g (7oz) mixed berries

4 x 120g (4¼oz) bags mixed salad leaves

1 x 200g (7oz) punnet mushrooms

1 onion

3 small oranges

4 orange peppers

2 parsnips

4 red onions

5 red peppers

198g (7oz) can salt-free sweetcorn kernels

1 bunch of spring onions

2 sweet potatoes

16 tomatoes

1 x 1.5kg (3lb 5oz) bag white potatoes

4 yellow peppers

Note: If you follow meal plans 1–3 week by week you may find that you have leftover ingredients that can be rolled over to the next week.

Dairy	Grains	Protein
1 x 220g (7¾oz) packet Cheddar cheese (reduced fat, if you choose)	1 small packet plain biscuits	12 eggs
1 x 500g (1lb 2oz) carton ready-to-serve custard	1 loaf wholemeal bread	400g (14oz) can low-salt/low sugar baked beans
1 x 200g (7oz) packet feta cheese	1 packet wholemeal pitta bread (freeze the ones you don't use)	2 x 400g (14oz) cans butter beans in water
1 x 1kg (2lb 4oz) carton Greek yogurt	2 x wholemeal rolls	2 x 400g (14oz) cans chickpeas in water
1 x 250g (9oz) packet mozzarella (reduced fat, if you choose)	1 packet wholemeal tortilla wraps	400g (14oz) can green or brown lentils in water
2 x 1kg (2lb 4oz) cartons natural yogurt		400g (14oz) can kidney beans in water
1 litre semi-skimmed or skimmed milk		1 whole chicken (about 1.2–1.5kg/ 2lb 10oz–3lb 5oz)
		1 x 80g (2¾oz) packet chorizo slices
		200g (7oz) dried red lentils
		1 x 400g (14oz) block firm tofu
		1 x 125g (4½oz) packet ham slices
		4 salmon fillets (400g/14oz in total)

Miscellaneous

1 x 30g (1oz) packet baked crisps

1 x slice of cake

1 x 160g (5¾oz) tub olives

1 x 190g (6¾oz) jar green pesto

Glossary

Alpha-linolenic acid (ALA): an OMEGA-3 FATTY ACID found in plant foods such as kale, spinach, seeds, nuts and oils.

Amino acids: the building blocks of proteins.

Antioxidants: vitamins, minerals or micronutrients that fight free radical damage in the body. Free radicals (unstable atoms or molecules) can cause harm leading to illness if their levels are too high.

Anthocyanins: ANTIOXIDANTS that give foods a blue/purple colour.

Atherosclerosis: a build-up of fatty deposits in the arteries.

Blood pressure (BP): a measure of how hard the blood is pushing against the artery walls.

Body mass index (BMI): a measure of an adult's weight in kilograms divided by their height in metres squared. This calculation is used to categorize your weight as normal/ overweight/obese, however there are other factors that can play a role.

Cardiovascular diseases (CVD): a general term for conditions that affect the heart or blood vessels. This includes heart disease.

Carotenoids: ANTIOXIDANTS that give food a yellow/orange colour.

Cholesterol: a type of fat found in the bloodstream and in the fatty outer layer of our cell membranes.

Deep vein thrombosis (DVT): a blood clot in a vein located deep inside your body, usually the leg.

DHA (docosahexaenoic acid): a type of omega-3 fat found in fish, shellfish and algae.

Diastolic blood pressure (DBP): the BLOOD PRESSURE when the heart relaxes and the ventricles are allowed to refill with blood.

Dietitian: someone trained in the science and medical research of nutrition. They have a legally protected title.

EPA (eicosapentaenoic acid): a type of OMEGA-3 FATTY ACID found in fish, shellfish and algae.

Essential hypertension (primary hypertension): high BLOOD PRESSURE due to unknown causes.

Fat-soluble vitamins: vitamins that dissolve in fat and are stored in tissue, so the body has access to them as needed. They comprise vitamins A, D, E and K.

Flavonoids: plant chemicals that have health benefits. They are found in a variety of fruits and vegetables.

Glycemic Index (GI): a relative ranking of carbohydrate in foods according to how they affect your blood glucose levels after eating.

HDL (high density lipoprotein): a type of CHOLESTEROL sometimes known as 'good cholesterol'. Higher levels are beneficial.

Hydrogenated: fully saturated with hydrogen molecules.

Hypertension (high BLOOD PRESSURE): a medical condition in which the blood pressure is consistently high.

Insoluble fibre: the roughage that keeps our bowels regular, found in the skins of fruit and vegetables, in the outer parts of wholegrains, and in seeds.

Insulin: a hormone that is released to help regulate the glucose levels in the bloodstream.

LDL (low density lipoprotein): a type of CHOLESTEROL that can raise your risk levels for heart disease.

Metabolic syndrome (or Syndrome X): a combination of diabetes, high BLOOD PRESSURE and obesity. This puts you at greater risk of coronary heart disease and stroke.

Monounsaturated fat: a heart-healthy dietary fat.

Normotensive: having or denoting a normal BLOOD PRESSURE.

Omega-3 fatty acid (omega-3 or omega-3s): a type of POLYUNSATURATED FAT where the first double bond is at carbon 3. The three main types are ALPHA-LINOLENIC ACID (ALA), EICOSAPENTAENOIC ACID (EPA) and DOCOSAHEXAENOIC ACID (DHA). They play an important role in human diet.

Omega-6 fatty acid (omega-6 or omega-6s): a type of POLYUNSATURATED FAT where the first double bond is at carbon 6. They play an important role in human diet.

Phytochemicals: plant chemicals with health benefits. They are found in fruits, vegetables, grains, beans, and other plants.

Plant stanols/sterols: plant compounds that can help reduce CHOLESTEROL levels. They are found in a range of plant foods such as cereals, vegetable oils, seeds and nuts.

Polyphenols: plant compounds with health benefits. They are found in fruits, vegetables, cereals, tea and coffee, and red wine.

Polyunsaturated fat: fats found in plant and animal foods that are usually liquid when at room temperature.

Pre-hypertension: a condition where the BLOOD PRESSURE is higher than normal, but not yet meeting HYPERTENSION.

Probiotics: live micro-organisms that feed the healthy bacteria in your gut.

Saturated fat: animal fats that are solid when at room temperature.

Secondary hypertension (secondary HIGH BLOOD PRESSURE): HYPERTENSION that is caused by another medical condition.

Soluble fibre: a type of dietary fibre that makes the stool softer, bulkier, more formed and so easier to move through the colon.

Systolic blood pressure (SBP): the BLOOD PRESSURE when the heart contracts and the ventricles push blood out to the rest of the body.

The DASH (Dietary Approaches to Stop Hypertension) trial: a piece of research carried out in 1997 by the DASH Collaborative Research Group to look at how eating a certain way may affect blood pressure.

Trans fats: a type of artificially created fat that can increase your LDL CHOLESTEROL levels and increase your risk of heart disease.

Triglycerides: a type of fat found in the blood that is formed of three fatty acids combined with a glycerol molecule. The body converts extra fat (that it doesn't use straight away) into triglycerides and stores them for later use.

Type 1 diabetes: an autoimmune disease characterized by the body's inability to produce enough insulin to regulate blood sugar levels, so these are too high.

Type 2 diabetes: a common condition where the body does not respond to the insulin that is produced, so there are high blood sugar levels.

UK Terms & Their US Equivalents

UK	US
aubergine	eggplant
baking tin	baking pan
baking tray	baking sheet
bicarbonate of soda	baking soda
butter beans	lima beans
cake tin	cake pan
caster sugar	superfine sugar
celery stick	celery stalk
chickpeas	garbanzo beans
chilli (fresh or dried), plural chillies	chile, plural chiles
chilli powder	chili powder
chilli sauce	chili sauce
coriander (fresh)	cilantro
cornflour	cornstarch
courgette	zucchini
dried chilli flakes	dried/crushed red pepper flakes
flaked almonds	slivered almonds
flapjack	oat bar/granola bar/ energy bar

UK	US
frying pan	skillet
grill (n)	broiler; grill (v) = broil
mangetout	snow peas
Marmite	yeast extract
mixed spice	apple pie spice
pepper (as in sweet red, yellow, etc)	bell pepper
pitta bread	pita bread
plain flour	all-purpose flour
rapeseed oil	canola oil
rasher (bacon)	strip (bacon)
rocket	arugula
self-raising flour	self-rising flour
sieve	strainer
spring onions	scallions
swede	rutabaga
tomato purée	tomato paste
wholemeal (bread)	whole-wheat

Endnotes

Introduction

1   PEN (2009). 'Using the DASH Diet to Help Lower Blood Pressure'.
    Dietitians of Canada.

2   Houston M. C. and Harper K. J. (2008). 'Potassium, Magnesium and
    Calcium: Their Role in Both the Cause and Treatment of Hypertension'.
    The Journal of Clinical Hypertension 10(7): 3–11.

3   Houston M. C. and Harper K. J. (2008). 'Potassium, Magnesium and
    Calcium: Their Role in Both the Cause and Treatment of Hypertension'.
    The Journal of Clinical Hypertension 10(7): 3–11.

4   NHS Website (2011). *Dukan diet 'tops list of worst celeb diets'.*
    Accessed 13/04/2020. <https://www.nhs.uk/news/food-and-diet/
    dukan-diet-tops-list-of-worst-celeb-diets/>

Chapter 1: Hypertension & the Heart

1   NHS Website (2018). *Cardiovascular disease.* Accessed 09/04/2020.
    <https://www.nhs.uk/conditions/Cardiovascular-disease/>

2   Challa H. J. et al (2020). 'DASH Diet (Dietary Approaches to Stop
    Hypertension)'. Treasure Island (FL): StatPearls Publishing [internet].

3   Siervo M. et al (2015). 'Effects of the Dietary Approach to Stop Hypertension
    (DASH) Diet on Cardiovascular Risk Factors: a systematic review and
    meta-analysis'. *British Journal of Nutrition* 113(1): 1–15.

4   British Heart Foundation (2020). *UK Factsheet.* Accessed 02/05/2020.
    <https://www.bhf.org.uk/what-we-do/our-research/heart-statistics>

5   Houston M. C. and Harper K. J. (2008). 'Potassium, Magnesium and
    Calcium: Their Role in Both the Cause and Treatment of Hypertension'.
    The Journal of Clinical Hypertension 10(7): 3–11.

6   Siervo M. et al (2015). 'Effects of the Dietary Approach to Stop Hypertension
    (DASH) Diet on Cardiovascular Risk Factors: a systematic review and
    meta-analysis'. *British Journal of Nutrition* 113(1): 1–15.

7   PEN website (2009). 'Using the DASH Diet to Help Lower Blood Pressure'.
    Dietitians of Canada.

8   National Institute for Health and Care Excellence (2019). *Hypertension in adults: diagnosis and management*. [NG136]. Retrieved from <https://www.nice.org.uk/guidance/ng136/chapter/Recommendations>

9   Houston M. C. and Harper K. J. (2008). 'Potassium, Magnesium and Calcium: Their Role in Both the Cause and Treatment of Hypertension'. *The Journal of Clinical Hypertension* 10(7): 3–11.

10 Public Health England (2020). *Hypertension prevalence estimates in England, 2017.* <https://assets.publishing.service.gov.uk/government/uploads/system/uploads/attachment_data/file/873605/Summary_of_hypertension_prevalence_estimates_in_England__1_.pdf>

11 Ozemek C. et al (2018). 'The Role of Diet for Prevention and Management of Hypertension'. *Current Opinion in Cardiology* 33(4): 388–393.

12 MacMahon S. et al (1990). 'Blood pressure, stroke, and coronary heart disease'. *The Lancet* 335(8692): 765–774.

13 Action on Salt website. *Blood Pressure*. Accessed 15/05/2020. <http://www.actiononsalt.org.uk/health-professionals/blood-pressure/>

Chapter 2: The DASH Diet – an overview

1   National Institute for Health and Care Excellence (2019). *Hypertension in adults: diagnosis and management*. [NG136]. Retrieved from <https://www.nice.org.uk/guidance/ng136/chapter/Recommendations>

2   Karanja N. et al (2004). 'The DASH diet for high blood pressure: from clinical trial to dinner table'. *Cleveland Clinic Journal of Medicine* 71(9): 745–753.

3   Sacks F. M. et al (2001). 'Effects on blood pressure of reduced dietary sodium and the Dietary Approaches to Stop Hypertension (DASH) diet'. *New England Journal of Medicine* 344(1): 3–10.

4   Ozemek C. et al (2018). 'The Role of Diet for Prevention and Management of Hypertension'. *Current Opinion in Cardiology* 33(4): 388–393.

5   Windhauser M. M. et al (1999). 'Dietary adherence in the Dietary Approaches to Stop Hypertension trial'. *Journal of the American Dietetic Association* 99(8 Suppl): S76–83.

6   Dyer A. R. et al (1994). 'Urinary electrolyte excretion in 24 hours and blood pressure in the INTERSALT Study: II. Estimates of electrolyte-blood pressure associations corrected for regression dilution bias'. *American Journal of Epidemiology* 139(9): 940–951.

7   Houston M. C. and Harper K. J. (2008). 'Potassium, Magnesium and Calcium: Their Role in Both the Cause and Treatment of Hypertension'. *The Journal of Clinical Hypertension* 10(7): 3–11.

8   Houston M. C. and Harper K. J. (2008). 'Potassium, Magnesium and Calcium: Their Role in Both the Cause and Treatment of Hypertension'. *The Journal of Clinical Hypertension* 10(7): 3–11.

9   Houston M. C. and Harper K. J. (2008). 'Potassium, Magnesium and Calcium: Their Role in Both the Cause and Treatment of Hypertension'. *The Journal of Clinical Hypertension* 10(7): 3–11.

10   Houston M. C. and Harper K. J. (2008). 'Potassium, Magnesium and Calcium: Their Role in Both the Cause and Treatment of Hypertension'. *The Journal of Clinical Hypertension* 10(7): 3–11.

11   Naini A. E. et al (2015). 'Effect of Omega-3 fatty acids on blood pressure and serum lipids in continuous ambulatory peritoneal dialysis patients'. *Journal of Research in Pharmacy Practice* 4(3): 135–141.

12   NHS Website (2019). *Metabolic Syndrome*. Accessed 17/06/2020. <https://www.nhs.uk/conditions/metabolic-syndrome/>

13   Siervo M. et al (2015). 'Effects of the Dietary Approach to Stop Hypertension (DASH) Diet on Cardiovascular Risk Factors: a systematic review and meta-analysis'. *British Journal of Nutrition* 113(1): 1–15.

Chapter 3: Getting Started on the DASH Diet

1   PEN (2009). 'Using the DASH Diet to Help Lower Blood Pressure'. Dietitians of Canada.

Chapter 4: Key Food Groups

1   Aune D. et al (2016). 'Whole grain consumption and risk of cardiovascular disease, cancer, and all cause and cause specific mortality: systemic review and dose-response meta-analysis of prospective studies'. *BMJ* 353:i2716.

2   Champagne C. M. (2006). 'Dietary interventions on blood pressure: the Dietary Approaches to Stop Hypertension (DASH) trials'. *Nutrition Reviews*, 64(2 Pt 2): S53–S56.

3   Institute for Health Metrics and Evaluation (IHME) (2017). *Findings from the Global Burden of Disease Study 2017.* IHME. Accessed 15/05/2020. <http://www.healthdata.org/sites/default/files/files/policy_report/2019/GBD_2017_Booklet_Issuu_2.pdf>

4   Public Health England (2020). *National Diet and Nutrition Survey: Assessment of salt intake from urinary sodium in adults (aged 19 to 64 years) in England, 2018 to 2019.* <https://assets.publishing.service.gov.uk/government/uploads/system/uploads/attachment_data/file/876624/Report_England_Sodium_Survey_2018-to-2019.pdf>

5   Tholstrup T. (2006). 'Dairy products and cardiovascular disease'. *Current Opinion in Lipidology* 17(1): 1–10.

6   Champagne, C. M. (2006). 'Dietary interventions on blood pressure: the Dietary Approaches to Stop Hypertension (DASH) trials'. *Nutrition Reviews*, 64(2 Pt 2): S53–S56.

7   Bernstein A. M. et al (2012). 'Dietary Protein Sources and the Risk of Stroke in Men and Women'. *Stroke* 43(3): 637–644.

8   Rohrmann S. et al (2013). 'Meat consumption and mortality – results from the European Prospective Investigation into Cancer and Nutrition'. *BMC Medicine* 11(63).

9   Craig W. J. (2010). 'Nutrition concerns and health effects of vegetarian diets'. *Nutrition in Clinical Practice* 25(6): 613–620.

10 Ha S. K. (2014). 'Dietary Salt Intake and Hypertension'. *Electrolyte Blood Press* 12(1): 7–18.

11 Public Health England (2020). *National Diet and Nutrition Survey: Assessment of salt intake from urinary sodium in adults (aged 19 to 64 years) in England, 2018 to 2019.* <https://assets.publishing.service.gov.uk/government/uploads/system/uploads/attachment_data/file/876624/Report_England_Sodium_Survey_2018-to-2019.pdf>

12 MacGregor G. A. et al (1982). 'Double-blind randomised crossover trial of moderate sodium restriction in essential hypertension'. *The Lancet* 1(8268): 351–355.

13 World Health Organization (2003). 'Diet, nutrition and the prevention of chronic diseases' Report of a joint WHO/FAO Expert Consultation. WHO Technical Report Series No. 916. <https://apps.who.int/iris/bitstream/handle/10665/42665/WHO_TRS_916.pdf;jsessionid=23204BA264D298D85DB8942E7BE1D462?sequence=1>

14 Ha S. K. (2014). 'Dietary Salt Intake and Hypertension'. *Electrolyte Blood Press* 12(1): 7–18.

15 Karanja N. et al (2004). 'The DASH diet for high blood pressure: from clinical trial to dinner table'. *Cleveland Clinic Journal of Medicine* 71(9): 745–753.

16 Sacks F. M. et al (2001). 'Effects on blood pressure of reduced dietary sodium and the Dietary Approaches to Stop Hypertension (DASH) diet'. *New England Journal of Medicine* 344(1): 3–10.

17 Ha S. K. (2014). 'Dietary Salt Intake and Hypertension'. *Electrolyte Blood Press* 12(1): 7–18.

18 Public Health England (2020). *National Diet and Nutrition Survey: Assessment of salt intake from urinary sodium in adults (aged 19 to 64 years) in England, 2018 to 2019.* <https://assets.publishing.service.gov.uk/government/uploads/system/uploads/attachment_data/file/876624/Report_England_Sodium_Survey_2018-to-2019.pdf>

19 BDA (2019). *Hypertension and Diet: Food Fact Sheet.* Accessed 13/04/2020. <https://www.bda.uk.com/resource/hypertension-diet.html>

Chapter 5: Lifestyle Advice

1 Redon J. (2001). 'Hypertension in obesity'. *Nutrition, Metabolism & Cardiovascular Diseases* 11(5): 344–353.

2 Mertens I. L. and Van Gaal L. F. (2000). 'Overweight, obesity, and blood pressure: the effects of modest weight reduction'. *Obesity Research* 8(3): 270–278.

3 Ozemek C. et al (2018). 'The Role of Diet for Prevention and Management of Hypertension'. *Current Opinion in Cardiology* 33(4): 388–393.

4 Blumenthal J. A. et al (2010). 'Effects of the DASH Diet Alone and in Combination with Exercise and Weight Loss on Blood Pressure and Cardiovascular Biomarkers in Men and Women With High Blood Pressure: The ENCORE Study'. *Archives of Internal Medicine* 170(2): 126–135.

5 BDA (2019). *Hypertension and Diet: Food Fact Sheet.* Accessed 13/04/2020. <https://www.bda.uk.com/resource/hypertension-diet.html>

6 Sisson S. B. et al (2010). 'Accelerometer-determined steps/day and metabolic syndrome'. *American Journal of Preventative Medicine* 38(6): 575–582.

7 Avila J. J. et al (2010). 'Effect of moderate intensity resistance training during weight loss on body composition and physical performance in overweight older adults'. *European Journal of Applied Physiology* 109(3): 517–525.

8   Valente E. A. et al (2011). 'The effect of the addition of resistance training to a dietary education intervention on apolipoproteins and diet quality in overweight and obese older adults'. *Clinical Interventions in Aging* 6: 235–241.

9   Karanja N. et al (2004). 'The DASH diet for high blood pressure: from clinical trial to dinner table'. *Cleveland Clinic Journal of Medicine* 71(9): 745–753.

Additional Reading Resources

Informedhealth.org [internet] (2012, 2019). *High Blood Pressure: Overview.* IQWiG (Institute for Quality and Efficiency in Health Care). Accessed 02/06/2020. <https://www.ncbi.nlm.nih.gov/books/NBK279239/>

Professor Frayn K. N. (Managing Ed.), BNF (British Nutrition Foundation), Stanner S. and Coe, S. (Eds.) (2019). *Cardiovascular Disease: Diet, Nutrition and Emerging Risk Factors.* Second Edition. (John Wiley & Sons Ltd, New Jersey).

Index

Recipe titles are in *italics*;
g = glossary entries

Acknowledgements

Thanks to my mum and dad, my biggest supporters, who taught me I can do whatever I set my mind to.

Thanks to my inner circle of friends, who have been there to listen to me as my writing progresses and have been a huge encouragement.

Thanks to my agent, Corrie, for her guidance and steady hand. Without her, I wouldn't have agreed to write this book.

Huge thanks to Octopus Books for commissioning this book and taking me through the process. It has been an unexpected joy to write, rooted in science and packed with the recipes I love.

Thanks also to my team of dietitian friends, who told me I could do this and were there with friendly chat when I needed it.

Author Biography

Priya Tew is an award-winning, experienced registered dietitian and winner of the British Dietetic Association's Media Spokesperson of the Year.

Her TV appearances include BBC News, Sky News, *Embarrassing Bodies, Food: Truth or Scare, Good Enough to Eat* and BBC One's *Eat Well for Less.*

https://www.priyatew.com/
https://www.pilateswithpriya.co.uk/